HAPPINESS

For more interviews and free resources head to:
HAPPINESS.info

Disclaimer:
This book is intended for educational purposes only. The opinions
presented reflect the research and ideas of the author or those whose
ideas the author presents, but are not intended to substitute for the
services of a trained health care practitioner. The author and the
publisher disclaim responsibility for any adverse effects resulting
directly or indirectly from information contained
in this book.

Hardcover: 978-1-7396491-0-4
Paperback: 978-1-7396491-1-1

First paperback edition August 2022.

Edited by Clara Abigail
Interior design by Asia Bizior
Cover art by Sangita Sutradhar
Author photo by Pablo Núñez Palma

Published by Claydon Hawke
ClaydonHawke.com

H

HAPPINESS

Well-Being Advice from the
World's Leading Experts

DUNCAN CJ

PRAISE FOR THE PODCAST

"What you're doing, this is very, very important. It would be at any time, but especially now."

GREGG BRADEN

5x *New York Times* bestselling author

"The world is a better place because of you and what you're doing."

ROCO BELIC

Academy Award-nominated director

"You have an incredible mind."

DAN SIEGEL, MD

5x *New York Times* bestselling author

"Keep doing what you're doing...It's wonderful."

MARK NEPO

#1 *New York Times* bestselling author
of *The Book of Awakening*

"(Duncan) is a phenomenally good student, young businessman, and wonderfully interesting and knowledgeable."

MARK VICTOR HANSEN

500 million books sold, $2B worth of branded products

"You really are good at this...you ask the right questions."

PAUL BLOOM, PHD

Award-winning researcher, Professor of Cognitive Science at Yale University

"Duncan, this is great...Thanks for
the good work that you do!"

STEVEN KOTLER

4x *New York Times* bestselling author

"Duncan, I loved our...connection and would
absolutely count you as a friend."

MO GAWDAT

Former CBO for Google [x], International bestselling author
of *Solve for Happy*

"You really knew what you were talking about.
Not everyone does."

SONJA LYUBOMIRSKY, PHD

Bestselling author of *The Myths of Happiness*

"Keep doing what you're doing."

JOHN RATEY, MD

Bestselling author of *Spark*, Globally-recognized pioneer
in neuropsychiatry

"Duncan CJ...the guy is the real deal."

MARK MATOUSEK

International bestselling author of *When You're Falling, Dive*

"Arielle Ford, Eric Edmeades, Sean Stephenson...
Greg Braden, Bruce Lipton, etc.!
We all agree that Duncan rocks."

DEBRA PONEMAN

Bestselling author

"You're an amazing man and a bright light on the planet."

MARCI SHIMMOFF

#1 *New York Times* bestselling author of *Happy for No Reason*

"What you are accomplishing with your vision... I'm honored to be invited to speak with you."

JOE QUIRK

President of the Seasteading Institute, Co-founder of Blue Frontiers

"That was fun!"

JOHN GRAY, PHD

The bestselling relationship author of all time, 50 million books sold.

"Duncan, a huge thanks to you."

CARL HONORÉ

International bestselling author, TED Speaker

"You can...really cause global change. I'm really glad we've met."

CHEN LIZRA

TED Talk, 10M+ views

CONTENTS

FOR

My parents, whose love and encouragement
have been a constant in my life.

And for all the incredible experts and thought leaders
in this book. You have been unbelievably generous
to me with your time and knowledge, and this
would never have been possible without you.
Thank you so much for teaching me, supporting
my work, and answering thousands of my questions.

WHY HAPPINESS?

I kiss my parents goodbye and watch as their car drives away. I've just arrived at my new school; it's a boarding school, so we sleep there. For anyone who isn't familiar with boarding schools, imagine Hogwarts minus the magic.

I'm thirteen years old. All my friends are in one house, but it's full, so I'm in a different one. I don't want to be in it, I don't know anyone here, but I'm trying to be brave.

I get changed into my new school tracksuit. Everyone in the school has the same uniform, which would make finding yours in the laundry a little tricky, but to avoid this problem, we all have name tags sewn onto the outside of our clothes. This would be fine except that my name is quite long, and we also ordered the wrong font size for the labels, so I have written in giant letters:

DUNCAN BYRON CAREW-JONES

Everyone has a study, and mine is on the second floor. These are just big enough for a desk and a chair. That's it. You can stretch out your arms and touch each wall, but the room is yours, and you can decorate it however you like. I unpack the two posters that I brought with me. One is black and white and is of Elle Macpherson – I put her on the right-hand wall. My second poster is in color and is of Kelly Brook. Kelly Brook is usually an English television presenter, but today she's in a field wearing a bikini. This is my favorite poster, so I put it directly above the desk. This is the best spot in the room – pride of place.

For the first few weeks, I spend most of my time alone. I don't have any homework to do, I don't have any friends to talk to, I can hear the sound of people playing football in the courtyard below, but I don't move.

Then I remember, there is one thing. I had discovered something pretty cool a few months earlier. I still don't understand how it works, but it's a lot of fun.

It doesn't have a lock, but I lean up against the door to stop anyone from coming in. I look up at Kelly, then at the bikini. I close my eyes, and I put my hand down my pants.

A few minutes later, I open my eyes, Kelly is still there, but not just Kelly – someone is climbing on the roof outside my window with a football in their hand.

They are looking at me and laughing.

I completely freeze.

I can't even take my hand out of my pants.

I look at him.

He's looking at me.

I begin pleading with my eyes.

*Please don't say anything…*Please!

My eyes are begging him!

And then he shouts, "*Busted!*"

"*Busted!*"

"There's a new kid wanking in his room!"

"Which one?" they call back to him.

He leans forward and reads the sign sown onto my chest.

"DUNCAN BYRON CAREW-JONES!"

That word...busted. I have nightmares about that word. People would come up to me and say, "Is it true you got busted?"

"Oi, Duncan, I heard you got wank busted!"

All day, every day, it's all I can think about. *Who knows? Do they know? Do those people know?*

If I'm in a group of people and one of them knows, I'd think, *Please don't bring it up. Please don't bring it up.*

Six months later, everyone in our school is excited about something. One of the older students has joined a boyband. And not just any boyband; they quickly become one of the biggest bands in England. They have four number-one singles; they sell five million records, are in every newspaper, and are on every television channel. I hear their name every single day for the next three years. *Everyone* is excited.

Everyone but me.

Because the name of the band is...*Busted.*

My parents know I'm not happy, and they're worried. I tell them it's because my friends are in a different house, and I don't get to watch much television, so I'm missing all of my favorite shows. Next time they come to visit me, they give me a card with a silly joke on the front of it, and then they hand me a parcel gift wrapped in brown paper with a ribbon on it. I open it and inside is a handheld TV. It has an antenna, and you can walk around with it.

I never tell them the truth about what happened because I'm ashamed.

But I could have, and they would have been kind to me.

Because that's the type of people they are, kind.

I ended up loving my time at school. I made some incredible friends and have so many happy memories. And as upsetting as it was at the time, the above memory is one of the things I'm most grateful for because I think it made me a nicer person. After that day, I always hated seeing people embarrassed or upset. I wanted to lift people rather than knock them down.

So, thank you to my parents for always showing me, through your actions, the power of kindness.

And thank you to Kelly Brook.

Well, first of all, Kelly, my apologies. This apology is twenty-one years late, but I'm sorry.

But also, *thank you.*

Thank you for making this book happen.

WHAT IS THIS?

For years, I've been fascinated by the question: Why are some people happy and others are not?

In 2014, I wanted to take my research to the next level, so I started a podcast called *HAPPINESS with Duncan CJ*. I began tracking down and interviewing the top thought leaders in the world. I spoke with people from a vast array of disciplines: from psychology to quantum physics, from business to pharmacology, from evolutionary biology to psychedelics.

I wanted people to have access to this information, to be able to learn how to improve their life and their mental state regardless of where they lived, their background, or whether or not they had any money.

People lead busy lives, and I'm assuming most don't have time to listen to hundreds of interviews, so I've tried to highlight the most powerful ideas in this book.

If you or anyone you love wants to know how to be happy, this is my attempt to answer that question for you.

READ THIS FIRST

EDITING

Since the beginning, my goal has been to present the experts and their ideas in their own words. I love the casual, back-and-forth feel of a real-life conversation, so I wanted to keep this. However, I've made some edits when necessary to help with the readability, for example, shortening some passages or adding a word or two to help with comprehension and flow.

TIME FRAME

The conversations in this book took place over eight years. Any references to time will not be accurate, so if an expert says, "In August of this year," the August they're referring to would have been a few years ago.

FOOD AND SLEEP

I'm not going to talk about nutrition or sleep in this book.

Not because I regard them as less important – the opposite.
I consider these foundations that need to be in place before
we start.

If you're exhausted or have an unhealthy diet, then life may seem
a lot bleaker. If this applies to you, go and have a sleep first, eat
something nutritious, and then we'll begin.

CHECKLIST

A few times per year, I used to get low, but I didn't know why; there was no reason.

Experiencing a loss – a death, a breakup – as upsetting as those things were, at least the pain made sense. I could point to something: "I feel sad because…."

But feeling down for no apparent reason scared me because if I didn't know why I was sad, then I didn't know how to fix it, and I didn't know how long the sadness would last.

When I first started the *HAPPINESS with Duncan CJ* podcast, I just wanted to be open and learn as much as possible about the science of happiness and fulfillment. For years, I resisted the temptation to draw conclusions or start compiling 'rules' or 'principles.'

I knew that if I did, I would run the risk of confirmation bias – the tendency to notice and draw attention to all the things that support one's claim and ignore or not even see all the contradictory evidence.

However, after spending years researching and interviewing hundreds of the top happiness and fulfillment experts on the planet, it became impossible to ignore certain ideas and principles appearing again and again and again.

I acted as a guinea pig and tested all the different lessons that I was learning to see how they would, or would not, improve my state.

Many things worked, but I only kept the best.

Eight laws of happiness that consistently make me feel good.

They had to be easy to remember; otherwise, I wouldn't apply them, so I created a simple checklist for myself with each concept starting with a different alphabet letter: A, B, C, through to H.

When I can answer 'Yes' to the eight items on my checklist, I am normally happy.

When I'm feeling off, frustrated, or down, I will go through the checklist in my head, and I'll realize that I've been neglecting one, or many, of the things.

When I was sad in the past, I often didn't know why, I didn't know how to fix it, and I didn't know how long it would last.

Now I have an answer to all three concerns:

1) Don't know why? I go through my checklist, and whichever thing(s) I am neglecting, then *that* will usually be why.

2) Don't know how to fix it? I focus on the things I am neglecting.

3) Don't know how long it will last? Now I do. Once I can answer yes to all eight things, my sadness usually lifts.

I AM...

APPRECIATING

BEING

CONNECTING

DIRECTING

EXERCISING

FORGIVING

GROWING

HELPING

APPRECIATING

I am focusing on what I'm grateful and thankful for.

BEING

I am taking time to slow down, be in the moment, be still or anything that counteracts my constant 'doing.'

CONNECTING

I am spending time with people I love and am giving these relationships the energy and attention they deserve.

DIRECTING

I feel like I'm the director of my own life. I feel a sense of autonomy and choice.
NB: This is not to be confused with a futile attempt to control life or an obsession with certainty.

EXERCISING

I am moving my body and being active.

FORGIVING

I am forgiving myself for things I did/didn't do, and I am forgiving others. I am releasing shame, secrets, and resentment.

GROWING

I am developing, progressing, and growing each day.

HELPING

I am helping others and contributing to something larger than just myself.

DAVID HAMILTON, PHD

PhD in Organic Chemistry, used to develop
drugs to treat cardiovascular disease
and cancer, bestselling author of *How Your
Mind Can Heal Your Body.*

*David used to work for a big pharmaceutical company;
his job was to build drugs to combat heart disease and
cancer. In the laboratory, he'd construct the drugs by
sticking atoms together. During this time, he became
captivated by the power of placebos. This fascination
led him to leave the industry and investigate how our
minds shape our bodies, health, and even our realities.*

There Are No Isolated Events

Duncan: If you take two people who share an emotional bond,
be it husband and wife, mother and daughter, you can do this
incredible test known as Correlations. What is this?

David: Science is funny because science is moving closer towards agreeing with the Tibetan Buddhist philosophy of emptiness, which says that everything is interconnected, deeply, at the
most fundamentally profound levels. Everything is connected,
and therefore, there is no separation between anything.

And one of the great experiments in science, not just quantum
physics but mainstream science that backs up that idea, took

people who shared an emotional bond. Let's say it could be husband and wife, mother and daughter, same-sex partners; it doesn't matter, as long as the people have an emotional bond. And one person goes in an MRI scanner, and the other's down the corridor. So, let's say, for argument's sake, it's a mother and daughter. So, the mother is in the MRI scanner. The daughter's down the corridor. She doesn't know that she's involved in the experiment, so she's just sitting in the waiting room, and all of a sudden, the scientist makes them jump. It's called the startle response, just like a little make-you-jump kind of thing, and at that moment of the daughter getting startled, the mother's brain picks up a flash in the visual cortex, which is the bit that processes visual information. And it's called the 'correlation' because what's happened is that the daughter has got startled… but the mother's brain registered it in real-time.

Duncan: And as you said, they're in different rooms, the mum didn't hear it, she didn't see it.

David: And these experiments are written up generally in science as 'correlations,' as you pointed out, between the neural states of people separated by a distance.

And it's almost like a scaled-up version of what people call quantum entanglement when you can take two particles – two paired particles – and separate them by the width of the universe, and if you pang one of them, the other one instantly feels it, so to speak. It's the same type of phenomenon, but we're seeing it on a large scale rather than just a quantum scale.

And that resonates very well with the Tibetan Buddhist's ideas of emptiness. They say that everything is interdependent at the deepest, most fundamentally profound levels, and everything depends on everything else. Nothing is isolated. Nothing is separate at all, fact.

Duncan: When you hear that study, what else does it make you think – what implications?

David: That everything matters. Our collective thoughts, our collective intentions. Not just our collective actions, but even small, seemingly insignificant things. There are no isolated events. That's what I would say: there are no isolated events.

Something that we feel is so insignificant – an exchange with someone down the street – you think is unimportant. There are no insignificant isolated events. Everything depends on everything else, and everything affects everything else.

And therefore, if we want to see, let's say, more fulfillment and happiness and peace in the world, we've got to be the source of that, we've got to start finding a way, not just being fulfilled and peaceful and happy ourselves but helping other people to have that kind of state.

And then what you see – because there are no isolated events, there are no individuals in that sense – then as we create that sense within ourselves and in our local environment, that *is* having a profound effect on the whole thing, on everything.

Kindness Makes Us Happier

Duncan: A side effect of kindness is happiness. Science has proven that kindness makes us happier.

David: Yeah. And it does it for several reasons. When you're kind, there's something emotional and spiritual that feels good, but neurologically, one of the things going on in the brain is that we're producing the brain's natural versions of morphine and heroin.

So just like getting high on drugs, you get a high out of connecting, out of being kind, and that explains what some scientists call "Helper's High," but it is a pharmacological high in the brain.

That's a side effect. But in the long term, numerous studies done in multiple different ways have all confirmed the same thing you said, Duncan, that kindness itself makes us happier, but the key is that it does it in the long term. If we're consistent with it, then happiness gradually increases in the long term.

Yeah, we get an instant hit from doing something kind because you feel good, you feel warm and connected to the person, there's a nice little feeling in the chest area. But if you do this consistently, not to gain from it but because it's the right thing to do, then what happens is your actual baseline happiness starts to increase.

Your deep sense of satisfaction is what gradually increases.

It's the consistency that's important with the kindness stuff.

Kindness Is Contagious

Duncan: And it's contagious. Kindness leads to more kindness. If you've done a kind thing to me, then I'm much more inclined to go and do a kind thing to somebody else. So even on the micro-scale, if you concentrate on being kind, you are changing a much bigger playing field.

David: Absolutely, there's no question that life itself is deeply interconnected. There are no isolated acts. On the deepest, more philosophical levels, every act of kindness is having an effect, is changing the world, if you like.

But on even the primary level, scientists at Harvard have measured this, how one act inspires another, and they've measured it goes out to three degrees of separation. What that means is when you randomly help someone, then chances are they will help someone else (one degree), who will help someone else (two degrees), who will help someone else (three degrees of separation). Three social steps – really cool!

So, if each person had four contacts, then you would find one act of kindness would affect four people, times four, times four, is sixty-four people.

And we don't realize the impact that the ordinary person has several times a day when you do something nice.

Paracetamol vs. Panadol

Duncan: Paracetamol and Panadol are the same. But what is the difference?

David: There was a study done a number of years ago, and it was on aspirin, and you can map the figures onto things like paracetamol, ibuprofen, and stuff.

Paracetamol and Panadol are the exact same thing, but you can buy paracetamol in the supermarket, certainly in the U.K., for 15p and Panadol's ten times the price. But because it's ten times the price, we have a little story in the head that says, "If something's more expensive, then it must be better," and we've heard it so many times, and we've had the direct experience of it. We've experienced paying more for an item of clothing, and it lasts longer. So, because we've taken that on board in a deep level in our minds when you buy a more expensive version of the same drug – you give it a different name and make the packaging all fancy, multiply the price by ten times – then it does work better because it's ten times the price.

But again, it's because of your mind, because you've taken an idea into your head that says, "If something's more expensive, then it must be better," and again, it's your mind that's making that work say ten, twenty, thirty or so percent better.

It's your mind that's doing it!

15th Leading Cause of Death in the U.S. = a Belief

Duncan: There's a very clever study a few years ago that looked at the link between stress and heart disease, but this study was different because they added a question to it. What was that?

David: If you do a study – and this is the kind of thing that's been done many, many times – you can draw a comparison between people's levels of stress over a long period.

So, let's say over ten years, people would monitor their levels. You could say how stressed you tend to be, and what you usually find is those who are more stressed tend to have the shortest life span.

And it's not something you see in day-to-day life as much, but over a population, statistically, what you tend to see is increases in stress tend to translate to more heart disease, therefore, shorter life span.

But in this particular study, they weren't just asking people, "What's your typical level of stress?" say, over the last period, but they asked them another question: "Do you believe that stress is bad for you?"

And it turns out that the belief itself made a world of difference because you had those people who were really stressed, and at the other end, you had those who were hardly stressed at all.

Amongst those who were really stressed but had the belief that stress was good for them, the death rate was lower than in those who were hardly stressed at all but who believed that stress was bad for them.

So, even if you've hardly any stress but believe it's bad for you, that's worse for you than having a lot of stress but believing that it's good for you.

When the scientists extracted the statistics, it turned out that the belief in stress itself was the fifteenth leading cause of death in the United States.

A belief! Not stress but a belief in stress made it onto the top twenty leading causes of death. A belief, a psychological thing – isn't that fascinating?

ERIC EDMEADES

Entrepreneur, international speaker, and creator
of transformational seminars, workshops,
and retreats worldwide.

*Eric is a serial entrepreneur. For over thirty years, he's
owned, run, started, and sold companies in a large va-
riety of industries. As a speaker, he's shared the stage
with Tony Robbins, President Clinton, and Sir Richard
Branson. A phrase I come across often is a quote by
Robbins, "The quality of your life is a direct reflection
of the quality of the questions you are asking yourself."
A quality question can be particularly impactful when
shitty stuff happens, like in Eric's story below.*

If I Had to Be Grateful About This, Why Would It Be?

Eric: How you view your past will color your view of the future.

Suppose you regard your past with anger, fear, resentment, hatred, and all these negative emotions. In that case, when you
turn around and look at the future, you will naturally assume
that your future will be full of negativity, anger, hatred, and
resentment.

And so, one of my fundamental core beliefs is the more grateful
you can become for your past, the greater faith you will have
in the future.

We did not come here to be bored.

Jim Rohn used to say, if you bought a book and the first chapter was boring, "Everything's going to be okay." You might read the second chapter, but man, if everything was still *okay* by the end of the second chapter, you're not going to finish that book.

Well, you didn't come here into this life for everything to be okay all the time. You didn't.

You came into this life for drama and experience and love and heartbreak and disappointment and elation, all of it! I don't even think you could taste joy if you didn't have disappointment. I don't think you'd ever really appreciate it.

If I can get to a place where I am grateful for everything that's ever happened to me, everything I've done or not done. If I can get to that place of absolute gratitude for my past, then when I turn around and I look to my future, I'm going to go, "Well, that doesn't look very nice, but I'll be grateful for it one day."

And I'll give you the perfect example of this. In August of this year, my wife and I arrived home. We stopped off at the grocery store to pick up groceries. We hadn't been home in six months. We had almost everything we owned with us because we'd been on tour for so long, traveling all over the world, working with people all over the world. We get home, and while we're shopping, the driver, who we knew, had some weird family problem, I suppose, and he arranged to have everything we owned stolen.

Everything.

I'd just spent a week with the Hadza bushmen with original photography. I had questions in from John Gray and Tony Robbins and all these incredible people who had sent me questions to ask the bushmen, and I'd done all these interviews on tape. All the video – gone! I'd just been with the chimpanzees of Mahale in Greystoke, wild chimpanzees. All these photographs – gone! Because it was just too much data to dump to the cloud from Africa. So, all these things are gone: laptops, gone; passports, gone; money, gone; clothing, gone; jewelry, gone. All gone!

So how do you feel? Anger, resentful – I did! I looked in the back of the truck, and I felt terrible. I was so full of anger and resentment, and then I stopped for a second, and I said, "Wait a minute now, how does anger or resentment help me at the moment?" If the guys were here right now, anger could be helpful, right? You know, adrenaline, anger, go beat somebody up, get my stuff back! But they're gone, so now there's no point, and my poor wife's over here, crying, upset, inconsolable.

And at that moment, I said to myself, "But you know, Eric, everything that's ever happened to you in the past, everything that you've ever regarded as an absolute calamity, ended up being the greatest gift." I had an employer completely scam me so badly once that I had to quit my job, we were living in a foreign country, and I thought it was the most terrible thing in the world, ended up being the most incredible gift.

When I was eighteen years old, somebody lit me on fire. They had to rebuild my arm from skin taken from my legs. I am so grateful that that happened. So, if I can be thankful for those things, maybe one day I'm going to look back on this empty van, and I'm going to be grateful that all of the stuff was stolen, and then my mind said, "No! No, you're not!"

Then I said, "No, maybe I am. But *if I was* going to be, why might it be?"

And I thought. I couldn't think of something.

And I was like, "No, no, no, but just think of one thing. What could you *one day* be grateful for about this event?"

And I said, "You know, I can think of one thing." Neither my wife nor me has a laptop, and it'll take two weeks to get replacement laptops because we use these super macked-out Macs, and I need to fly to New York to go get one because we lived in the Caribbean. I had two weeks without a laptop. You know what? That's going to be good for our relationship. We're going to hang out, go for more walks on the beach than we usually do, nice dinners out, we'll cook more because we don't have our computers to distract us and be working all the time, and I thought, you know that's going to be pretty cool. Plus, we'll get to do a lot more kiteboarding than we usually do because I have all this work to do, and now I can't do it. And then also my wife, her Mac is, like, three years old, she won't let me buy a new one for her, and I'm her I.T. director, so I have to fix it. So now I get to buy her a new Mac!

Then finally, I had this big realization that, holy crap, if this had happened to us five years ago, it would have been heartbreaking because we had put a lot of money into a company we bought. We were in deep financial trouble, and if we'd lost forty thousand dollars worth of stuff, passports, and everything back then, it would have been soul-destroying. And I'm like, thank God it happened now! And by the end of this whole conversation, I started going:

I'm going to get to buy my wife all new clothes, that's going to be great!

I'm going to buy myself a new Mac.

I've got this going on.

We're going to go kiteboarding all week.

I started going, *This is wicked!*

Duncan: Haha.

Eric: You know what? I've wanted to live without a cell phone, I've wanted to experiment with life without a cell phone for ages, but I've never had the discipline. Now my phone is gone, and I'm not buying a new one. Awesome!

By the way, I lived for six and a half months without a mobile phone after that. Six and a half months, no mobile phone. I wrote an eighty-thousand-word fiction book with no effort. I got more done in the following six months after all our stuff got stolen than I got done in the previous two years. And I got a glimpse of that as I was looking into the back of the van. And so I turned to my wife, and I said to her, "Everything's going to be okay."

And she said, "What do you mean, everything's going to be okay? All our stuff is gone."

And I said, "Let me tell you right now, with confidence, with certainty, I can tell you everything is going to be okay. You and I are about to have the funnest two weeks we've had in a whole long time, I promise!"

And she stopped crying. And she started to feel better. And then we had the best two weeks you could imagine.

And then I wrote a book, and then I got more work done than I could imagine, and we're having the most incredible year in our business because I had six months of a completely different perspective.

> **Note**: *Eric told me this story five years ago, and since then, whenever I've received upsetting news or been struggling with something, I'll ask myself that question: "If I had to be grateful about this, why would it be?"*
>
> *And then I'll continue asking and answering it again and again.*
>
> *Without fail, it has transformed my mood and my perspective.*

There Is No Certainty

Duncan: Certainty. Why is it so important to let go of the need for certainty?

Eric: First of all, it's an illusion. There is no certainty. There is no certainty of anything.

This is probably getting clichéd at this point; I've been saying it for years and years, and so have others, so I think it'll be a cliché soon enough. But you are right now sitting on a rock that's rotating at an incredibly high speed and whipping through space at sixty-five thousand miles per hour, and there are comets all over the place.

And when you look at a picture of the solar system, and it looks all neat and tidy with the planets, you should take a look at the solar system with all the cosmic dust and materials and rocks in it, and you'd realize it's a crapshoot out there, man!

We exist through the grace of the right accidents happening every single day. What I'm getting at is that certainty is already an illusion.

And so, when we become attached to certainty, what that makes us want to do is hold onto things. And when you hold onto things, you can't move.

> **Note**: *So much unhappiness is caused by people stressing and worrying about things completely out of their control.*
>
> *Trying to control something you don't have control over is a lousy use of your time.*
>
> *According to Mo Gawdat, who we'll meet later on in the book, there are only two things that you have complete control over, your actions and your attitude.*

"The need for certainty is the greatest disease the mind faces."

ROBERT GREENE

"I was in a state of constant suffering, and it took me years of rejection, anger and frustration to see the light and accept the truth: *I wasn't in control.* When I realized that, I felt a ton of weight removed from my shoulders. My actions remained committed, but my attachment to outcomes completely vanished... Take the responsible action first, then release the need to control."

MO GAWDAT

JOHANN HARI

One of the most-viewed TED Talkers of all time,
bestselling author of *Lost Connections:
Uncovering the Real Causes of Depression –
and the Unexpected Solutions.*

*Johann has come onto the podcast on two occasions.
Each time we ended up chatting for far longer than the
planned thirty minutes, so this profile is longer. The second time we spoke was unique. The interview was about
to begin when I heard a scream from the next room.
I go to investigate. Oh dear, there's a cobra in my house.
And we didn't see where it went. It's hiding in the room
somewhere, but we're not sure where. Luckily for me,
I was about to interview one of the top anxiety experts
in the world. Much of what I know today about depression and anxiety is because of Johann. His research can
improve the lives of millions of people. I recommend
people check out his book Lost Connections.*

Isolation Is a Catastrophe

Duncan: Professor Sheldon Cohen carried out this study which
you talked about where he took a bunch of people and recorded
how many friends and healthy social connections each of them
had. With their permission, he then put them in contact with
the common cold virus.

And the isolated people were three times more likely to catch a cold than those who had healthy social connections. That was fascinating.

Johann: Professor Martha McClintock did this study with rats and found that isolated rats are something like eighty times more likely to develop the rat equivalent of breast cancer than rats living in connection with other rats.

Isolation is a catastrophe for a social species.

One of the reasons why the Amish have such low levels of depression and anxiety is because there are no isolated Amish. There is plenty to criticize about the Amish – I'm a gay atheist, you can imagine I'm not a big defender of the Amish – but there's no loneliness there.

The Opposite of Addiction Is Not Sobriety

Johann: The theory of addiction we've got about chemical hooks – that chemical hooks cause drug addiction – comes from a series of experiments done earlier in the twentieth century. They're simple experiments.

You take a rat, put it in a cage, and give it two water bottles. One is just water, and the other is water laced with either heroin or cocaine. The rat will almost always prefer the drug water and almost always kills itself within a couple of weeks. So, there you go, that's our story!

But in the seventies, Professor Bruce Alexander came along and looked at these experiments and said, "Well, hang on a minute, you put the rat alone, in an empty cage, where it's got nothing to do except use these drugs. What would happen if we did this differently?"

So, he built a cage called Rat Park, which is basically like heaven for rats. They've got loads of friends, loads of cheese, loads of colored balls, they can have loads of sex, anything rats like, and they've got both the water bottles, the normal water, and the drug water. And of course, they try both; they don't know what's in them.

This is the important thing: in Rat Park, they don't like the drug water, they almost never use it, none of them ever use it compulsively, none of them ever overdosed.

So, you go from almost a hundred percent overdose when their lives are shit; they're isolated, they don't have the things that give life meaning, to none, when they have the things that make life meaningful.

And I think this has a lot of lessons for humans. There have been a lot of human experiments on this principle, and I guess the way I've tried to distill it is to say: The opposite of addiction is not sobriety; the opposite of addiction is connection.

We Have Deep, Underlying Psychological Needs

Johann: For me, one of the key moments was when I interviewed a South African psychiatrist called Dr. Derek Summerfield, and Derek happened to be in Cambodia when chemical antidepressants were first introduced there in 2001. And the local doctors, the Cambodian doctors, didn't know what these drugs were, so he explained to them, and they said, "Oh, we don't need them, we've already got antidepressants."

And he said, "What do you mean?" He thought they were going to talk about some herbal remedy. Instead, they told him a story.

There was a farmer in their community who stood on a landmine and got his leg blown off. So, they gave him an artificial limb, and he went back to work in the rice fields. But apparently, it's extremely painful to work underwater when you've got an artificial limb. I imagine it was quite traumatic as he's been blown up there. He starts to cry all day; he doesn't want to get out of bed, classic depression.

Doctors said, "Well, we gave him an antidepressant."

Derek said, "What was it?"

They explain that they went and sat with him, they listened to him, they realized that his pain made sense. It wasn't some irrational malfunction; it had perfectly understandable causes. They figured if they bought him a cow, he could become a dairy farmer; he wouldn't be in this situation that was upsetting him so much. They bought him a cow. Within a couple of weeks, his crying stopped. Within a month, his depression was gone. They said to Derek, "So that cow, that's an antidepressant, that's what you mean, right?"

If you've been raised to think about depression the way we have, that sounds like a really bad joke: "I went to my doctor for an antidepressant; he gave me a cow." But what those Cambodian doctors knew intuitively is what the World Health Organization, the leading medical body in the world, has been trying to tell us for years: if you're depressed, if you're anxious, you're not a machine with broken parts.

You're a human being with unmet needs, and you need love and support to get those needs met.

Everyone listening to this knows they have natural physical needs. You need food, and you need water, you need shelter, you need clean air. If I took them away from you, you would be in terrible trouble.

There's equally strong evidence that human beings have natural psychological needs. You need to feel you belong; you need to feel your life has meaning and purpose. You need to feel that people see you and value you. You need to feel you've got a future that makes sense. There's a whole range of them. Our culture's good at many things, I'm glad to be alive today, but we've been getting less and less good at meeting these deep, underlying psychological needs. And it's certainly not the only thing that's going wrong, but it's a big factor in why we have this growing depression and anxiety crisis.

What's the Antidepressant for Loneliness?

Duncan: Being deeply lonely causes as much stress, as much cortisol, as being physically attacked by a stranger.

Johann: Yeah, there are a few things about this. We are the loneliest society that's ever been in the Western world. So, to use the outlier – the U.S. – there's a study that asks Americans, "How many close friends do you have who you can call on in a crisis?"

Years ago, when they started doing it, the most common answer was five. Today, the most common response is none. It's not the average, but it's the most common answer.

One of the people who taught me so much about this, a man called Professor John Cacioppo at the University of Chicago, the leading expert in the world on loneliness, recently died. Just a devastating loss because he was a relatively young man, and he made so many breakthroughs in his field. He was the person who discovered what you just showed – that cortisol, the stress hormone, we release as much of that when we're acutely lonely than when we're punched in the face by a stranger.

And Professor Cacioppo made all sorts of incredible breakthroughs about loneliness. He proved that it causes depression and anxiety. And his argument for why, I found quite persuasive.

Duncan, why are you and I alive? One key reason is that our ancestors on the savannahs of Africa were really good at one thing – they weren't bigger than the animals they took down in a lot of cases, they weren't faster than the animals they took down. They were a lot better at banding together in groups and cooperating.

Just like bees evolved to need a hive, humans evolved to need a tribe.

And this is deep in our deepest ingrained impulses.

If you were separated from the tribe, you were depressed and anxious for a good reason: you were probably about to die.

That was a signal to get back to the group as quickly as possible.

We know that loneliness has massively increased, and I wanted to figure out, well, what's the antidepressant for that? It turns out there is one.

One of the heroes of my book is a man called Dr. Sam Everington. Sam is a doctor in East London, where I lived for a long time, in a poor part of East London. Sam's a general practitioner, a GP. And he was uncomfortable because he had loads of patients coming to him with depression and anxiety, and he'd been told in his medical training – even though he knew this wasn't true – to say to people, "You've just got a chemical imbalance in your brain," that's all that's going on, and just drug them. Like me, Sam's not opposed to chemical antidepressants, he thinks they do have some role, but he could see it wasn't solving the problem for most of them. And he could see one of the problems they had was they were really, really lonely. So, he decided to pioneer a different approach.

One day, a woman came to him called Lisa Cunningham, who I got to know well. Lisa had been shut away in her home for seven years with crippling depression and anxiety. Sam said to

Lisa, "Don't worry, I'll carry on giving you these drugs, but I'm also going to prescribe something else. I'm going to prescribe you to take part in a group." There was an area behind the doctors' surgery known as 'dog shit alley,' which gives you a sense of it. It backed onto a park, though. And Sam said to Lisa, "What I want you to do is come and turn up twice a week. I'll turn out and support you. I want you to meet with a group of other depressed and anxious people, and together, we're going to turn dog shit alley into something beautiful."

The first meeting they had, Lisa was physically sick with anxiety.

Several things happened. The first was the group had something to talk about that wasn't how terrible they felt. Normally, we either drug depressed people or give them an opportunity to go and talk about their pain, both of which have value, but this was something else. They decided they were going to learn gardening. They decided they were going to put their fingers in the soil. They were going to learn the rhythms of the seasons.

There's a lot of evidence that exposure to the natural world is a powerful antidepressant.

So, they started to interact with the natural world and began to learn something they didn't know. These were all inner-city Eastenders – they didn't know anything about these things.

Another thing that happened was they began to form a tribe, and they did what human beings do when we form tribes: they started to solve each other's problems. So, for example, there was a guy in the program who was sleeping on the bus, the night bus. Everyone was like, "Well, of course, you're depressed if you're sleeping on the bus." They started to pressure the local authority to get him housed, and they succeeded; they got him a home. It was the first time they'd done something for someone else in a long time. It made them feel great.

The way Lisa put it to me: "As the flowers began to bloom, as the garden began to bloom, we began to bloom."

There was a study in Norway of a very similar program, part of a growing body of evidence that found it was more than twice as effective as chemical antidepressants.

I think for kind of obvious reasons, right, it was dealing with two of the key reasons why they were depressed and anxious in the first place: their disconnection from other people and their disconnection from the natural world.

And I saw this all over the world from Sydney to Sao Paulo to San Francisco – the strategies that dealt best with depression and anxiety were the ones that dealt with the reasons why we feel so bad in the first place.

Nature Deprivation

Johann: The state prison in Michigan – just by coincidence, no one designed it this way – has one part that looks out over beautiful greenery and another part that looks out over a parking lot, a concrete parking lot, and it's random where you end up in the prison.

The people who look out over the lush greenery developed thirty-three percent fewer mental health problems than those who looked out over bare concrete.

We know that animals in zoos go crazy when they're deprived of their habitat. Parrots rip out their feathers, horses start obsessively swaying, and so on.

A similar thing happens with humans when we're deprived of our natural habitat. Nature deprivation makes us depressed.

Happiness for Me or Happiness for Us?

Johann: I interviewed this amazing woman called Dr. Brett Ford. She's a social scientist at Berkeley (now at the University of Toronto). With her colleagues, she did this fascinating research. So what they want to figure out is if you consciously and deliberately decided you were going to try to be happy – "I'm going to spend two hours a day trying to make myself happier." – would you become happier?

And they did this research with their colleagues all over the world, in four countries: in the U.S., in Russia, in China, and Japan. And what they found was fascinating.

In the U.S., if you try to make yourself happier, you do not become happier. But in the other countries, if you try to make yourself happier, you do become happier.

And they were trying to figure out, well, why is that? What's going on? So they did all sorts of breakdowns of the research. And what they saw when they did the analysis was, in the U.S. – and I'm pretty sure this is true in Europe, although perhaps to a lesser degree – if you try to make yourself happier, generally you do something for yourself:

- You buy something.
- You show off on Instagram.
- You try to get a promotion.

In the other countries, if you try to make yourself happier, generally – these are averages, not in every instance – generally, you try to do something for someone else. You do something for your friends, your family, your community. So, they have an instinctively collective idea of what happiness is, and we have an instinctively individual idea of what happiness is.

And it turns out our idea of happiness – which is instilled in us by this machinery of advertising and deep aspects of our culture – doesn't work very well. A species of individualists would have died out on the savannahs of Africa; we're not that species.

But these collective ideas of happiness do work to a much greater degree.

And again, that helps us to understand why there's been this big rise in depression and anxiety at the same time as a rise in individualism.

THE NEWS

Newsstand magazine sales increase by around thirty percent when the cover is negative instead of positive. And a "good news day" resulted in a decrease in readership of sixty-six percent in an online Russian newspaper.[1]

This makes sense; our heightened interest and focus on danger and threats is what kept our ancestors alive.

However, this feature has turned into a bug. There aren't saber-toothed tigers around every corner, but we still have the same ancient software running our modern lives. Evolution is *slow*.

There's a saying in the media: "If it bleeds, it leads."

"I've worked in the newspaper, so I know what happens in the news zone. You're basically told, 'Find the thing that's going to scare people the most and write about it.'...It's like every day is Halloween at the newspaper. I avoid newspapers, I avoid web surfing," says entrepreneur and bestselling author James Altucher.[2]

The cognitive psychologist Steven Pinker writes, "The nature of news is likely to distort people's view of the world because of a mental bug that the psychologists Amos Tversky and Daniel Kahneman called the Availability heuristic: people estimate the probability of an event or the frequency of a kind of thing by the ease with which instances come to mind. Plane crashes always make the news, but car crashes, which kill far more people, almost never do. Not surprisingly, many people have a fear of flying, but almost no one has a fear of driving. People rank tornadoes (which kill about fifty Americans a year) as a more common cause of death than asthma (which kills more than four thousand Americans a year), presumably because tornadoes make for better television."[3]

An analogy that I liked was told to me by a real estate investor called Daniel Latto. He asked me, "Where do you get your beliefs from?"

I replied, "Family, from society, the news, the media...."

He cut me off and said, "Think about the news for a second – do you want to be getting your beliefs from the news? And what's the news? The news is that one journalist, an editor, one chief of programming have decided that this is the story we're going to run today. And that's gone through his filters. If you were in a warehouse, a very dark warehouse, and you had a small torch, and you shone your torch in the corner, and let's assume there's a party going on in this warehouse, and you shine your torch in this corner, and two people are having an argument. You would go away and go, "Well, that's a terrible party," if that's what you're looking at, but actually, everyone else is having an awesome time. That's the news."

I'm not suggesting that people bury their heads, that they are ignorant to what is going on in the world, or that they avoid many of the unpleasant realities of life.

Not at all.

But is having minute-by-minute updates of all the worst examples of human nature making you more informed?

Or is it forming in you a picture of the world that is both inaccurate and harmful?

We live in the attention economy.

More attention = more advertising revenue = higher profits.

So, unless something really awesome happens, like your country wins the World Cup, it makes more sense for media companies, financially, to play to our base human fears and anxieties:

Murder! Terrorism! Recession!

Financial meltdown!

Flu epidemic!

Be scared!

Our brains have something called a reticular activation system (R.A.S.). Think of it like Google but for the brain. When we type something into Google and click 'Search,' it shows us results that it believes are relevant.

In the same way, when we focus on something, our brain starts to 'search,' and it shows us results that it believes are relevant.

If your focus is that *people are dishonest.*

Then, no problem! It can find countless examples to show you.

If your focus is on *everything wrong with your partner, relationships, job, etc.*

Then, easy! It can fill libraries with examples and evidence to support your claim.

However, if your focus is *all of the things you have to be grateful for.*

Then, also easy! It will fill your life with a never-ending flow. You will see evidence everywhere you look.

"If I know everything about your external world, I can only predict ten percent of your long-term happiness. Ninety percent of your long-term happiness is predicted not by the external world but by the way your brain processes the world."

SHAWN ACHOR

MARCI SHIMOFF

Transformational leader, one of the bestselling female nonfiction authors of all time, author of *Happy for No Reason: 7 Steps to Being Happy from the Inside Out.*

My interview with Marci finished. She turned to me and said, "Do you have any advice for what I can do better next time 'round?" It wasn't just lip service; she wanted to know. At the time, I'd been around for a few years but was unknown in the industry. Marci had sold millions of books. She once had three titles on the New York Times bestseller list simultaneously, but she wanted to hear my feedback. This stuck with me, and I found it inspiring. I've since learned that many of the happiest and most fulfilled people are lifelong learners.

The Negativity Bias and How to Reverse It

Marci: The average person has sixty thousand thoughts a day, and eighty percent of them are negative.

Duncan: Eighty?

Marci: Eighty percent for the average person. We inherited this. Psychologists call it the negativity bias. It's our tendency to focus on the negatives more than the positives and to remember them more. And we inherited that from our caveman ancestors who needed to remember the negatives, or they would die.

But we no longer need that habit of holding onto the negatives.

A dear friend of mine, a brilliant colleague named Rick Hanson – he wrote a fabulous book called *Buddha's Brain* – and Rick says our minds are like Velcro for the negative – the negatives stick to us – but they're like Teflon for the positives – the positives slide off of us.

I'll give you an example. If you get ten compliments in a day and one criticism, what do you remember at the end of the day?

Duncan: The one criticism.

Marci: The one criticism.

First of all, don't beat yourself up for having it because it's a natural thing. These are neural pathways that are in the brain.

But happier people reverse that tendency.

There are three things to do:

Number one, you've got to be on the lookout for the positive. Look out for it. One of the women I interviewed says she pretends she's on the Academy Awards Committee, and every day, she's looking out to give five Academy Awards. So, she sees a little cute, white, fluffy dog walking in the park, and she goes, "Oh, that dog gets the cutest dog of the day award." So you're just training your mind to be looking out for what's good.

The second thing is you've got to savor it for at least twenty seconds for the good to start creating new neural pathways in the brain. So, the process of writing it down that's causing you to focus on it for more than just a couple of seconds.

And then the third thing the scientists say is to go for the three to one ratio, three positives to one negative. Now that's not so easy to do, but that reverses this old habit pattern, and over time, you'll notice a difference.

A great happiness researcher, Robert Emmons from the University of California, Davis, researched this gratitude practice that you were talking about. At the end of the day, write down three to five things during the day that you were grateful for, and within one month, it's shown to raise your happiness level.

Ho'oponopono

Marci: I'm often asked the question, "What's the one most important thing you can do to be happy?" And I think that's similar to what you've just asked, and there are many things that I could say, but the most important thing you can do to propel yourself forward is forgiveness. Forgive! Forgive everything. And forgiveness doesn't mean condoning. Forgiveness means that you're freeing yourself from the burden of anger or resentment. The person could be gone, they could be dead, it doesn't matter, and some of it is self-forgiveness.

I will tell you my favorite forgiveness tool or technique that I use. There are lots out there, but my favorite one is so simple. It's called *ho'oponopono*. It's based on a Kahuna Hawaiian tradition, which is why there's all those Os and Ps in it; you never have to be able to say the word *ho'oponopono*. It's four phrases that you repeat internally in your heart, and they are:

I'm sorry.

Please forgive me.

Thank you.

I love you.

And it doesn't matter who's right, who's wrong. You just feel those phrases towards the person or situation you have problems with and towards yourself.

Do we have time for me to share a story about how I've used this in my life?

Duncan: One hundred percent.

Marci: So, I've used this a million times, but the time that was the most powerful and significant to me was almost six years ago. My sister and I had gotten into an argument, and we weren't talking. And this had never happened in our family, and it was tense, and we went about four months without talking.

One morning, we all gathered to move our mother from our family home of fifty-eight years to an assisted living apartment, and we were all getting together to unpack her things. And I was so nervous because it was the first time seeing my sister when we hadn't spoken, and I walked into the apartment, and I hugged and kissed everybody hello except her. She and I ignored each other. She was off in the kitchen unpacking. We went through the whole morning ignoring each other, and you could feel the tension in the air. You could cut it with a knife. It was awful.

And after about three or four hours of this, I couldn't take it anymore, so I left, and I went to my car to meditate and just take a break, and I remembered ho'oponopono. So, I sat in my car, and I did that towards her. I just felt towards her:

I'm sorry.

Please forgive me.

Thank you.

I love you.

And towards myself as well. And I did that for about five minutes, and I suddenly felt this wave of love come over me. I realized that my sister wasn't mad at me for what had happened four months earlier, but it was a lifetime of stuff. And for the first time, I got it, and I got it from her point of view, and I felt so much love and compassion for her that I felt flooded with love.

So I went back into the apartment, and I decided not to say anything to anybody. I just went back in and continued unpacking my mum's things, and not more than three minutes of me being back, my sister came over to me, totally out of the blue, grabbed me by the hand, and said, "Come on, Marci, let's go unpack mum's closet together," which is what we did. An hour later, we're at lunch. My sister hands me her baked potato and says, "Marci, you have mine; you like these more than I do." And I was so shocked by this sudden change in her that I pulled my brother aside and I said, "Okay, what did you say to her?" and he said, "Marci, no-body's said anything, we have no idea what has just happened."

Well, Duncan, that was the beginning of an entirely new relationship that I now have with my sister, and thank God it happened when it did because nine months later, my sister and I found ourselves standing in that same closet of our mother's. But this time we were packing up Mum's things because she had just died unexpectedly. And thank God we had had that healing.

I say this story because I know that everybody listening has someone in their life that they need to do some more forgiveness with, or even yourself; it may be yourself.

And so again, I invite you, don't take my word for it, but try this out as an experiment and see what happens. I have heard thousands of stories from people who have used this and have just had amazing results, so try it out.

"If we could read the secret history of our enemies, we should find in each [person's] life sorrow and suffering enough to disarm any hostility."

HENRY WADSWORTH LONGFELLOW

"To accuse others for one's own misfortune is a sign of want of education. To accuse oneself shows that one's education has begun. To accuse neither oneself nor others shows that one's education is complete."

EPICTETUS C.55 AD – AD 135

DACHER KELTNER, PHD

Professor of Psychology, bestselling author, founder and director of the Greater Good Science Center, author of *Born to Be Good: The Science of a Meaningful Life.*

'Dog eat dog,' 'every man for themselves,' greed, selfishness. There is a lot of messed-up stuff in the world, but I'm an optimist despite this. I believe in humanity, and I think humans – at their core – are compassionate and kind. But maybe I'm wrong? Perhaps I'm being naive and kidding myself. I wanted to investigate what the research had to say. There was one man I needed to speak with: Dacher Keltner.

Human Beings Are Born to Be Good

Duncan: When you wrote the book *Born to Be Good*, one thing that you became acutely aware of was actually how good human beings are. In light of everything that's going on at the moment, you turn on the news, the politics, that's quite a reassuring thing. This is what your research told you, that human beings are essentially good?

Dacher: Yeah, and it is a very timely thing to remember today with everything that's going on. In the past thirty years or so, there's been this big shift in evolutionary thinking where we've realized that we're a very caring species; we care for vulnerable offspring. We're a very empathetic species compared to our primate relatives. We know what others feel and really imitate a lot. We are a very collaborative and cooperative species; we're able to work together on just about everything.

And then for me, Duncan, what all of those shifts translate to is that we have these amazing, what Adam Smith called 'moral sentiments,' things like compassion, gratitude, awe, wonder, that really help us build up strong societies, and what that tells us, for people who are struggling today with Brexit in England, the rise of right-wing political movements in other parts of Europe, in the United States, is that we have these very powerful, old tendencies that I think can countervail those more base sides to human nature.

Duncan: Oxytocin. Why is this such a special chemical?

Dacher: When you say that you're born to be good, like the title of my book, that's a strong claim because it says we have these innate tendencies to be kind or to share, what have you, and then what that further posits is that we should have physiological systems in our bodies and chemicals that help us be good to each other.

And my lab's worked very assertively on that thesis, and one of the most amazing of the chemicals that help us be good to each other is this little neuropeptide called oxytocin. It's produced in your brain stem. It goes up into your brain, and then it also floats through your blood, and it goes to tissues and target organs in your body. Oxytocin is involved when mothers give birth. It's involved in milk let down when Mum's see their babies and get, "*Oh, it's so cute,*" and it's covered in the post-birth fluid and stuff. That's oxytocin tricking the mum into being good to that thing.

And studies, time and time again, show it helps us connect to, cooperate with, and share with other individuals who we feel are part of our tribe. There are controversial findings right now about whether it helps us connect to people who are really different from us, and the evidence is mixed there, but it really does open us up to be good to others.

Duncan: The fact that it's survived for millions of years of evolution, is it fair to say it's got a massive evolutionary benefit?

Dacher: Yeah, it does. So we know it's important for humans to cooperate, be it in taking care in the evolutionary sense of our vulnerable offspring or cooperating in food gathering or the like.

And studies show that if I take a little whiff of this oxytocin with a nasal spray, I share more with you. If I'm in a romantic partnership, I forgive you, and I don't have as much conflict with you. It's amazing.

And we, in our lab, have traced levels of oxytocin back to particular genes – for example, on the sixth chromosome that influences how much oxytocin you have circulating in your body – and those genes predict more empathy and openness to others. So this is one of the most direct pieces of evidence for the thesis: we've evolved to be good.

Greed Machines or Sharing Machines?

Duncan: The idea that got popularized by Gordon Gekko (in the film *Wall Street*), the philosophy that "greed is good" has become internalized. Many people believe this. How dangerous do you feel that belief has been to our societies?

Dacher: Thank you for asking that, Duncan. Science is very useful when it can lead to evidence that challenges our basic ideas.

In the United States and many parts of the world – I suspect in parts of London, India, Beijing, Dubai – there is this idea that we are designed as greed machines – to maximize our self-interests.

And you know, it's funny, I've been teaching the science of happiness both at Berkeley and then on an online platform, and the data disconfirms that notion.

A) For the individual, if I pursue materialism and greed, I become less happy, and studies show that time and time again, it's more important to prioritize experiences or connections with people.

B) We know if I pursue greed, I create unequal social structures. And we know that unequal social structures make people less happy.

We know that healthy people balance; they balance self-interest with other-interest.

That Gordon Gekko statement drives me nuts!

There are studies now of Felix Warneken at Harvard University showing that eighteen-month-olds will share stuff intuitively; they'll help people in distress.

Most people are inclined to share.

Duncan: If that is the more intuitive thing and the greed is the part reinforced by the media or society, then, if that's our nature, it's hopeful that we can return to a more sharing, compassionate way.

Dacher: Very much so, Duncan. Another study is very telling on this, which is this work by David Rand at Yale, where he gave people the opportunity to share resources with a stranger. If people made the decisions fast and intuitively, they shared a lot. They shared over fifty percent of the resource. But if you asked them to think about what they should do, all of a sudden

Western culture seeps into their mind, and they're like, "What did I learn in that economics class?" and "What was that speech by Gordon Gekko?", oh yeah, *I should keep stuff for myself*, and they shared less.

So, I think what that tells us is we have these deep intuitions, and then from my perspective, we need to refashion culture to make it more sharing. One in five people in the United States are in poverty; they're hungry. That shouldn't happen, so we need to share more.

I take heart. I think that's what's happening with your generation. Younger folks in the United States are more interested in sharing; they're more oriented towards a better society. They're more skeptical like you of the Gordon Gekko thesis. My generation just said, "Oh yeah, greed is good."

I think we'll see shifts as your generation takes power.

MOST MISUNDERSTOOD
SCIENTIST OF ALL TIME?

On page after page of the ignored writings that complete Darwin's theory, he describes how "the moral qualities" primarily drive human evolution, much more than natural selection.[4]

The evolutionary systems scientist Dr. David Loye writes, "What Darwin actually believed and...wrote out at length has been twisted by a century of economic, political, and scientific "business as usual" to lock in the *exact opposite* of his original intention. Today the focus is mainly on Darwin's *Origin of Species*. But in the 828-page sequel in which he tells us he will now deal with *human* evolution, *The Descent of Man*, Darwin writes only twice of "survival of the fittest," but 95 *times of love*. He writes of selfishness 12 times, but 92 *times of moral sensitivity*. Of competition 9 times, but 24 times of mutuality and mutual aid."[5]

Dr. Ervin László is a systems scientist who has published more than seventy-five books and has twice been nominated for the Nobel Peace Prize, and he describes Darwin and his work as "one of the most cited yet also most misunderstood scientists of all times."[6]

"Darwin believed that love...is the prime mover in human evolution."

RAYMOND TREVOR BRADLEY, PHD

DUNCAN GOOSE

Founder of the One brand and Water Unite, over $25M donated, 3.8M lives changed, winner of European Entrepreneur of the Year.

I went to a TEDx event in 2014, and one of the speakers that stood out to me was a man called Duncan Goose. He was a down-to-earth and unassuming guy. But he was doing extraordinary things. He and his team were transforming the lives of not hundreds, not thousands, but millions of people. I was keen to learn more about his life, so we sat down for a virtual chat a few weeks later.

The Kindness of Strangers

Duncan: You said, "I was fortunate to have people all around the world take me under their wing when things went wrong as they sometimes did, and I learned a lot about humanity and the kindness of strangers."

Duncan G: Yeah, I think this was – I just got chills while you said that – I think it was possibly the greatest revelation for me.

Up until that point, I'd been living in London, and I lived in a street of terrace houses. I didn't know more than, like, one neighbor each side of our house, of a road that was probably about a hundred houses or something like that, and yeah, when you step outside this country, suddenly the level of interest that people have in you and wanting to help you is just – it's mind-blowing.

So, I'll give you a couple of examples of that, if I may. The first one was that I started on the east coast of Canada in Nova Scotia and was riding across the country. But a couple of weeks into that trip, I hit a deer early in the morning at about fifty, sixty miles an hour, and I ended up down a ditch, and the deer was dead, and the bike was a complete mess. It was not a great start to what would be a 'round the world trip. But the ambulance crew that picked me up and the police were phenomenal. The nearest hospital was an hour's drive away, so it was pretty re-mote where I was, but this community just came around me when they found out here was this foreign guy who'd hit a deer and come off his bike, and it was a mess. And they patched my motorbike up with Ski-Doo parts because there was no motor-bike shop where I was, but there were Ski-Doos. They stitched all my clothing back together, and they offered me a cottage to stay, and people took me out to ice hockey games when I was recuperating. It was just the most – it was like having this family around you that were just there, and it was an incredible and very humbling experience.

And then the other one was that I was motorbiking through Pakistan from Amritsar on the Indian border, right up in the north, down to Iran, and all of the way through Pakistan, no-body would let me pay for food. It was just amazing, and I don't know where that level of hospitality comes from, and there was a guy there who fixed my motorbike for me because I'd had some problems with it.

If anybody listening to this picks out anything from anything that we talk about, it would be to go out into the world and meet people because it's a phenomenal place. It's full of incredible, incredibly generous people.

BERNIE SIEGEL, MD

Retired pediatric surgeon and bestselling author of *Love, Medicine and Miracles: Lessons Learned about Self-Healing from a Surgeon's Experience with Exceptional Patients.*

One of my first-ever podcast guests was Dr. Bernie Siegel. I was still trying to figure out how to conduct a good interview. I never gave my guests any time to think. I would ask long, meandering questions that never got to the point and I began most sentences with the word fantastic. But none of these things was a problem with Bernie. We were about fifteen minutes into the interview, and I still hadn't asked a single question. Bernie did not need questions. Questions are for rookies. Bernie told me a story – which reminded him of a cool study – which reminded him of another story. I sat back in my chair, relaxed, and thought, fantastic.

Do Your Parents Love You?

Bernie: Harvard students were asked, "Do your parents love you?" Some said no, some said yes, and then they looked them up thirty-five years later. Of those who said yes, twenty-four percent had suffered a major illness in the intervening years. Of those who said no, ninety-eight percent had suffered a major illness.

If you go into assisted living – I work with a lot of seniors too – and you say, "Did your parents love you?" They look at you like you're nuts. "Of course they did."

They're eighty and ninety years old, and I always say to them, "You wouldn't be sitting here if they hadn't loved you," because what you do to yourself if you don't feel love…to make up for the fact that you didn't get love…food, alcohol, drugs, you're always looking for something to feed yourself, and then you hurt your health.

The Power of Hope

Bernie: There was a chemotherapy program with four drugs. They began with the letters E, P, O, and H. It was called the EPOH protocol. One of the doctors noticed that if you turn it around, it spells *hope*. He gave *hope*, but the others continued to give EPOH. They were all providing the same treatment because this was a study.

He had seventy-five percent of his patients respond. They had twenty-five percent.

And I saw that in the office too. I realized people believed what I said; it's hypnotic. A simple example: I did, as you mentioned, children's surgery. I'd say to the parents, get a bottle of vitamins but put a new label on it, whatever's bothering your child – hair-growing pills, anti-nausea, etc. – and whenever your son says, "Oh, my stomach doesn't feel good."

"Here! This will take care of it."

"Want your hair to grow? Take this pill every day!"

And it was amazing, and if any nurses are watching this, take an alcohol sponge when you're going to draw blood and tell the person, "This'll numb your skin; it's a new kind of sponge so you won't feel the needle." A third of the people will be hypnotized by it and say, "That's wonderful." Others will say, "I felt it, but it's a different level." "I felt it, not 'Ahh, oh that hurt,'" and by doing that, especially with kids, they wouldn't get all frantic if they saw the needle and would expect that, "Oh, it's not going to hurt, that's okay, go ahead."

One more simple example. In the emergency room, I was just in the habit of trying to reassure the children that were going off to surgery, and I'd say, "You'll go to sleep when you go in the operating room." I'm thinking of anesthesia, you know, trying to take away their fear. And it began to be just a laughing matter because the kids would fall asleep when we wheeled them in.

Duncan: Before the anesthesia?

Bernie: Yeah. Everybody in the operating room would start laughing because the kids would flip over, turn on their side, and they'd go out. And then they'd get mad at me for putting them on the operating table and waking them up. That was the funniest part; they'd start yelling at me, "You said I'd sleep."

I Love You; I Don't Like What You're Doing

Bernie: I always say you don't have to like what is going on, but love the person.

I love you; I don't like what you're doing.

Those are two separate things. And then people can listen to you, knowing that you care, but that you're trying to make their behavior safer or more caring, and so forth.

SEAN STEPHENSON

(1979-2019) Therapist and Doctor of Clinical Hypnosis, shared the stage with U.S. Presidents and the Dalai Lama, bestselling author of *Get Off Your "But": How to End Self-Sabotage and Stand Up for Yourself.*

Sean was born with a rare disorder that stunted his growth. It caused his bones to be very fragile (more than two hundred fractures by the age of eighteen). Despite his challenges, he spent his life helping others, inspiring millions of people during his twenty-five-year speaking career, and appearing on places like the Oprah Winfrey Show and Jimmy Kimmel Live! The Biography Channel produced a one-hour feature on his life called 'Three Foot Giant.' The more time I spent studying happiness, the more I came across a common belief, something that was sabotaging the lives and joy of millions of people: the belief that 'I'm not enough.' Sean spent his life researching insecurity, so I wanted to speak to him about this.

How to Keep Insecurity Dormant

Duncan: You think that insecurity is something that never completely goes away, don't you? But when we realize what it is, we can stay ahead of it. We can surround ourselves with the right people, the right environments.

Sean: Absolutely. So, insecurity, in my opinion, and from my research, is that feeling that you're not enough.

And when you don't feel like you're enough – I'm not tall enough, I'm not smart enough, I'm not wealthy enough, I'm not attractive enough, I'm not powerful enough, confident enough – whenever you feel like you're not enough, then you start to go down in a downward spiral and your decisions, and your choices, and your belief systems, everything starts to swirl around that "I'm not enough," and that's the root of the insecurity.

I went on a long journey to figure out how to get rid of insecurity – how do we pull it out of us?

Duncan: How do we banish it once and for all!

Sean: Right. How do we kill it? Thinking like a guy, how do we assassinate this!

Whereas, I found that you can't. You can't get rid of insecurity. All you can do – and you already alluded to it – is you can stay ahead of it, you can keep it dormant, and the way you keep it dormant is through great self-care. That when you take good care of your mind, your body, your spirit, when you're exercising, you're eating right, you're hanging out with positive people, you're listening to great programs like this, you're immersing yourself in an environment and a set of daily routines and rituals that build you up, then your insecurities, they don't flourish, they don't surface to run the show.

And that's just how I've seen it. If I could find something else that would be better than that, I would be talking about it, but everything I've found that said it was going to eliminate insecurity that wasn't based on that was just a parlor trick, and it didn't last. I've got a doctor in hypnosis, I've got a background as a trainer of NLP, I've gone to *so many* different courses where I was either told or hinted at that this was going to get rid of your insecurities. And what I've found is it helped, it certainly didn't hurt having any of the techniques that I've learned, but they were all temporary.

The only thing that lasts is putting yourself in an emotional and physical environment that nurtures you and is a part of self-care.

Duncan: This is something I've heard about for years, but recently every single book, audio, TED Talk, everything I'm reading, I come across again and again and again, "You are the average of the five people you spend the most time with," or "Your network is your net worth," or just any spin on the same theme.

The people you surround yourself with are the people you become.

Sean: And it's something that I am still, to this day, even though I'm writing the books and teaching this stuff, I'm still having to put into practice. Every year that goes by, I probably have to take out one or two people in my network that have just become toxic. Maybe they're not negative, but perhaps they're scarcity-driven, or they're underhanded; they're not above board in how they live their life. And it pains me to eliminate them because I may love them, I may care about them, but when you let a toxic behavior continue to be a part of your existence, you start to take it on yourself.

Never Believe a Prediction That Doesn't Empower You

Duncan: You said, "Never believe a prediction that doesn't empower you."

Sean: Well, it's actually drummed up a lot of upset in people, which is interesting.

You're going to be given a lot of labels throughout your life. You're going to be given labels that are empowering, and you're going to be given labels that are disempowering. And the reason why my mentality has always been "Never believe a prediction that doesn't empower you," is because if you're given the prognosis of death, let's say, early in your life, [Sean received this prognosis], what good does it serve you to believe that?

Because if you are going to die, then just believing you're going to die is only going to accelerate the process as well as pull down your spirits.

If you are going to die but don't want to believe that, you have a fork in the road. Maybe you end up dying, but you go out feeling strong and like you did your best.

Or you actually recover, and your will and your imagination and your determination cause a bend in what everybody thought you were going to be headed for. Now you're on a new trajectory because of that attitude – because of refusing to believe that negative prediction, you survive now.

All the analysts, doctors, and experts say it was a quote "miracle," it was "spontaneous," and meanwhile, you know it's because you didn't believe that pessimistic prediction.

And it upsets people because ever since I said that on that TED Talk, I've read thousands of comments from people around the world saying, "That's ridiculous, you have to believe negative predications or your life can go in all kinds of crazy directions." My mentality is, "No, no, you don't!"

Somebody says, "This business is not going to work," "Your body's not going to survive," "This relationship can't work."

When you start believing in other people's fears, it becomes so difficult to navigate your own life.

I believe that it's hard enough to navigate your own fears; you cannot let into your mind other people's. Because then you're just going to be bombarded with the world's fears, and that's going to stop you from going after what you want.

Common Form of Self-Sabotage = One Bucket

Duncan: You're a doctor, you're a therapist, you've worked with thousands and thousands of people. What self-sabotaging things or recurring themes do you see coming up again and again?

Sean: What people will do often is they will gravitate towards what they are successful at.

Let's say they struggle in business and love, but they are good at hitting the gym, and they work out every day and have an incredible body and put all their time and attention into their body. But meanwhile, they're lonely, and so after they go to the gym and build bigger muscles, they drink themselves to sleep because they're lonely and they have no one to love, and no one to love them.

So, some of the self-sabotage is pouring all your attention and energy into one bucket instead of making sure that you're working on all of them.

See, I Knew It! I'm the Chubby Kid!

Sean: Imagination, that inner image, as Dr. Maxwell Maltz in *Psycho-Cybernetics* talks about, that inner image drives us.

If somebody thinks of themselves as the little chubby kid and now they're forty-five years old, and they're like, "I'm always going to be the little chubby kid," then it doesn't matter how much weight they lose; internally, they still feel like that chubby kid.

And it's only a matter of time that they're going to want to prove that that's who they are, so they'll fall off the diet, slowly stop exercising, and then they're back to gaining the weight and think, *See, I knew it! I'm the chubby kid!* And that's because the human brain is equipped with a 'right machine.'

We want to be right.

And the question is: what do we want to be right about?

I want to be right about being a world thought leader that gets the human race to stop being so insecure and start acting from other spaces.

And so, therefore, I take actions, and I see that, and I work on it, and when I get down and out, I have to remind myself, "No, you're a world thought leader, get back up, the world needs you," and that imagination has to be sparked because willpower is not enough on its own – it burns out.

"The outer conditions of a person's life will always be found to reflect their inner beliefs."

JAMES ALLEN (1864 –1912)

THE STRONGEST
FORCE IN THE HUMAN
PERSONALITY

TONY ROBBINS

"Human beings absolutely follow through on who they believe they are. If you said to me, 'Well, I'm really going to work hard to stop smoking, but you know I've been a smoker my whole life, and I'm, you know, I am a smoker.' I know your days are numbered. You're going to be back smoking cigarettes again because we all act consistently with who we believe we are. I tell people the strongest force in the whole human personality is this need to stay consistent with how we define ourselves... Often, we made decisions in our youth or very young about what to believe, about what we were capable of, about who we are as a person, and that becomes the glass ceiling...that controls us."[7]

30 DAYS OF FEAR

It was three years ago. I've just moved to Amsterdam. I don't know anyone yet, so I spend each day exploring and walking up and down streets for hours. Despite being new in town, I've already found my secret spot. It's this tiny cafe tucked away down a narrow lane. It's warm and cozy, and they do the best sandwiches.

The place has a Dutch name, but the English translation is 'The Last Crumb.'

I'm sitting in this cafe reading a book. I see a gorgeous girl walk through the door and join the queue. I want to talk to her. I want to ask her out, but I don't know what to say.

Screw it, I get up and join the queue; I'll figure it out in the moment. I lean forward to make it look like I'm reading which sandwiches are on the menu. *Just say something*, I think, *Anything.*

"Excuse me, do you know what type of cheese Manchego is?"

It's not the best start, but she's about to answer when the man from behind the counter says, "Ahhhh, Manchego, Manchego,

Manchego. Manchego is a slightly creamy cheese. It's stronger than your average cheddar, but it's not too powerful."

I thank him.

The girl smiles and turns around.

She orders something and then sits down.

I pretend to order and then go back to my table where I already have a sandwich.

I try to think of a new plan.

You don't need a plan; she's almost finished her sandwich, go and say hi.

I don't move.

Ask her whether you can take her for a drink at some stage.

I don't move.

I want to.

But I'm scared.

I do nothing.

I watch her stand up, hand her plate back to the person behind the counter, and walk out.

———

"That's never going to happen, ever again!" I say to my roommate. "For the next thirty days, I will ask someone out *every* day! No phone, no apps. Just walking up to people. Face to face. In fact, not just people on their own. I want it to be even harder – they have to be in groups. At least fifty percent of the people I ask out have to be surrounded by friends, so I embarrass myself not just in front of one person but in front of an entire crowd."

I'm in a park; I see a girl. I walk up to her.

"Hi, my name's Duncan. Ermm, I was just wondering whether… Errr, sorry, I was just wondering whether, not like now, necessarily, but at some stage, or *maybe* now, if you want, it can be now, but it doesn't *have to* be now… I could maybe buy you a drink?"

As the last words leave my mouth, I realize that she's holding onto a man's hand.

I'm asking her out while she's holding her boyfriend's hand.

A girl is cycling next to me.

"Hello," I say.

"Hi," she replies.

"How are you?" I say.

"Good," she says. "It's my birthday!"

"Happy birthday! Would you like to go out with me?"

"Sorry?" she says.

"Would you like to go out with me?" I repeat.

"Erm, sure…"

"Great. What's your number?"

Her bike starts turning left.

"Looking forward to it," she says.

"But you never gave me your number?" I say.

"Okay. I'll see you there!" she says.

"Where?" I call after her as she cycles away. "*Where?*"

I'm in a restaurant called Coffee and Coconuts. I walk up to a table of people having lunch and start to ask one of them out. As I do, I see that her hand is rubbing her belly.

I look down and realize that she's *at least* nine months pregnant.

I have a dilemma: do I stop asking or continue?

I don't want her to think that she's not attractive because she's pregnant.

Also, it's the twenty-first century; maybe it was a one-night stand?

Maybe she's a widow?

Or perhaps she's a surrogate?

I decide to continue.

She laughs in my face, then points towards her hand and the wedding ring.

Today, the fear of failure, embarrassment, and rejection is still there, but it's weak; it's lost all its power.

A few months ago, I was walking around Amsterdam. I see a girl with long brown hair having a cigarette outside a building. She's wearing jeans, a denim jacket, and has headphones on.

She is stunning. I want to ask her out.

So, I take a deep breath and walk up to her.

She says yes.

And then she says, "I recognize you."

"Oh yeah, where from?" I say.

"I'm not sure," she says. "I'm not sure."

I tell her that text messages have recently stopped working on my phone, so she sends me a Facebook friend request. Then we say goodbye.

I look at her profile, and as I'm clicking through a few of the images, one photo catches my attention. It's from a couple of years ago. She's sitting in the corner of a tiny balcony, and the caption reads, "My secret spot."

I recognize it.

The place has a Dutch name.

But the English translation is 'The Last Crumb.'

CAL NEWPORT, PHD

Computer Science professor at Georgetown University, bestselling author of *Digital Minimalism: Choosing a Focused Life in a Noisy World.*

What do many university commencement speeches have in common? If you listen to lots of them, you'll start to hear the same piece of advice. Follow your passion. That is the key. Passion, passion, passion. But is this recommendation helpful? The person who has investigated this topic more than anyone else I know is Dr. Cal Newport.

Why 'Follow Your Passion' Is Bad Advice

Duncan: From the 1980s onwards, people have been convinced that we *all* have a passion that is an intrinsic trait, like our eye color or height. And that career happiness is simply a matter of introspection.

We do our introspection, we discover what our passion is, we find a career that matches that passion, and *then* we will be happy!

What is wrong with this?

Cal: Yeah, this is an issue I tackled in a book I wrote back in 2012 called *So Good They Can't Ignore You*, where the whole idea of the book was to understand how people end up loving what they do for a living. So, it's a simple premise: let me go study people who love what they do for a living, let me look at the research literature, let me try to get a clear answer to this question, "If you want to end up loving your work, feeling satisfied, feeling happy, what do you do?"

And the very first thing I found doing this research is that the most dominant answer is what you said. "It's all about matching your work to a preexisting passion, that you have some inborn, innate passions that if you can identify them through introspection and match them to your work, you will love what you're doing for a living. If you get the wrong match, on the other hand, you won't love what you're doing for a living, so the most important thing you can do is introspect and match!"

This hypothesis, this theory, this strategy falls apart under any analytical scrutiny.

This idea that we have preexisting passions and matching that to our work will make us love our work doesn't hold up if you look into it. And there are two significant flaws with it.

One: It assumes that most people have clear, preexisting passions that you can identify and use as the foundation of career choices. Most people don't! And we don't have evidence that this is common, especially for young people. This idea that you're just going to find, through introspection, some career preference that happens to match what the existing economic landscape and job opportunities happen to be at this moment in time is just sort of nonsense.

In fact, we have quantitative evidence that says, especially for young people, clear, preexisting passions are very rare. So, if you're telling people, "Follow your passion, follow your passion, it'll be fine." Most people don't have passions; that advice is incredibly counter-productive. It's impossible to follow if you don't have a clear preexisting passion.

The second problem is that it assumes if you really like something, and then you match that to a job, you'll really like the job.

We don't have a lot of evidence that it's true. Think about all the clichéd stories of the passionate amateur baker who opens a bakery and is miserable. Those clichés alone are enough to tell us that what leads to satisfaction in someone's work is much more complicated than "I like this subject, and now my job involves this subject, I will now really like my job."

It's more complicated than that. It has to do with autonomy and mastery and connection and impact and creativity.

Creating a job of passion and satisfaction is more complicated than that simple storyline would tell us. And the point I've been making in that book and beyond it is: it's worth embracing that complexity.

"You're meant to do something; if you can find out what that is, you'll love your job." We have to get past that simple idea, that sort of Disney movie plotline, that slogan, and embrace the complexity of how people build satisfaction in their careers. Because once you embrace it, you have a good chance of getting there!

What Leads to Job Satisfaction?

Duncan: You mentioned autonomy, impact, mastery, connection. What would be a better approach, say, you're good at something, it's not necessarily your passion, but you're good at something. Then you add being autonomous. You add that it makes an impact. You add a sense of mastery to it. Are you then much more likely to *love* that thing? Is that the approach that you would recommend?

Cal: Yeah, so here's the way I would think about it. So, as I mentioned, the research is pretty clear that the type of things that make people really satisfied in their jobs, make them find passion in their work, are those traits we just mentioned, like having a real sense of autonomy, you're in control over what you do and why you do it; having a sense of mastery, you're very good at something that the world values and you get that clear feedback; for a lot of people, connection, connection to peoples, connection to communities, connection to what it is that they're serving; and a sense of impact as well can be very, very important.

And for a lot of people, a sense of creativity, not for everyone, but a lot of people, the feeling of "I'm creating something new from scratch" can be very fulfilling.

Those five elements are not tied to specific types of work. So the key to passion and satisfaction is not finding *the right job*. The key to passion and satisfaction is getting as many of those elements as possible into your working life.

And many, many different types of careers, many, many different types of fields can provide those things. The match is not what's important; it's getting those specific work agnostic traits.

So, the question is, how do you get autonomy or mastery or impact into your career?

It's helpful to think about it in economic terms. Those traits are very desirable. Many people want them in their job, so there's a market for them; they're valuable traits. Therefore, if you want them, you have to have something valuable to offer in return.

Do you want a lot of autonomy in your career? Do you want a sense of mastery? Do you want real impact or creativity? Those are very valuable; they're scarce. If you want them, you need something valuable and scarce to be able to offer in return.

The marketplace of jobs does not care that "Hey, I'm passionate about this," or "I'd really, really love a job where I have all these things, can't I have one now, please?" It's a little bit more competitive than that.

"Okay, if you want these things, what do you have to offer that's rare and valuable in return?"

So, what you see if you study people who love what they do is they almost always begin with this apprenticeship phase, where they are honing rare and valuable skills that the marketplace unambiguously values.

They then use those skills as their currency to acquire in their career traits like autonomy, a sense of mastery, a sense of impact, and a sense of creativity. They make a financial transaction: "I've built up these valuable skills. I'm now going to take them out for a spin."

And how am I going to do that?

I will use them as leverage to get these good traits into my career.

Satisfaction, passion, fulfillment then grows along with those traits coming into their career.

So that's the much more consistent path to passion, fulfillment, and satisfaction in your career. Build up unambiguously rare and valuable skills. Then use those skills as leverage to shape your career around the attributes we know make people passionate.

And this is a very different storyline than simply, "You were born to be a sports social media marketer, and once you know that, if you can then get that job, you're set, and you'll be happy going forward!"

DUANA WELCH, PHD

Former Professor of Psychology, known for using social science to solve real-life relationship issues, author of *Love Factually*.

Our emotional and physical environment has a significant impact on us. We learned earlier how the people we spend the most time with are the people we become; this made me think about our love life and the romantic partners we choose. We often receive relationship advice from the people closest to us, but what does the data say?

What Healed a Heartbreak?

Duncan: What are some of the common mating myths that you come across repeatedly, that every time you hear, you're like, "No, that's not true!"

Duana: Yeah, oh, that's a great question, Duncan. So a big one is, "I've just come off a bad breakup, so what I need now is to be alone," or someone recently said to me, "I need to walk the earth." Eighty percent of my clients are men, which may surprise some of your listeners and viewers today. But there is this idea that we have to be strong and independent and that needing somebody else is weak and that you can only have a healthy relationship after you've got all your ducks in a row. And science is just really against that.

So, one of the more interesting studies on this to me is one done by a developmental psychologist named Mavis Hetherington. And Dr. Hetherington was studying people who are getting a divorce. A severe loss, this isn't just a breakup; this is a breakup of such proportions that children are involved, whole families are involved, communities are involved when you get a divorce.

And so she interviewed the two people who were getting a divorce, interviewed their children, and then interviewed any new partners they had, every year, for twenty years. Incredible stuff, really great science.

And what she found was that none of the following things helped people get over their heartbreak, none of them. It didn't help if you got more religion. It didn't help if you approached your guru. It didn't help if you got more therapy. It didn't help if you spent all your time alone. It didn't help if you spent all your time with friends. The thing that helped people reintegrate was none of the things that people tell you will help. Do you know what it was?

Duncan: I want to know.

Duana: Getting into a happy relationship with another person.

We need love in our lives.

The idea that we get better before we can have a good relationship is the reverse of what is real. What is real is we get better and do better after we're in a happy relationship.

65 Years of Relationship Science in One Sentence

Duncan: You said, if you had to summarize over sixty-five years of relationship science in just one sentence, it would be, "If you can find a partner who is kind and respectful and you are kind and respectful also, then your love life will probably go really well. If you can't, it won't."

You can't get more straightforward and in-a-nutshell than that. Kindness and respect on both sides, and you're already the majority of the way there?

Duana: Yeah, that does summarize the research.

Do No Harm but Take No Shit

Duncan: Do no harm but take no shit.

Duana: Yeah, that turns out to be my motto, Duncan. It has transformed my life. Kindness and respectfulness do not mean living a life without boundaries; you must be kind and respectful to yourselves also.

And that means no squatters' rights. People don't have the right to be in your life simply because they have been there. They must be treating you well to earn their place.

So, do no harm, go out of your way to do good, but don't accept what you wouldn't tolerate if it were happening to your best friend or your parents or your child or someone else you care about. Have standards that are loving to you.

MO GAWDAT

Former Chief Business Officer for Google [X], founder of the movement One Billion Happy, bestselling author of *Solve for Happy: Engineer Your Path to Joy.*

One person making a significant positive impact in the world is Mo. His personal story is powerful; his happiness mission is inspiring. And he knows how to explain hard-to-grasp ideas in a way that is clear and accessible.

An Equation for Happiness

Duncan: If the events in our life meet our expectations, we feel happy. If the events in our life miss our expectations, we feel unhappy. Is that right?

Mo: Yeah, so the equation was important for my research. As an engineer, a lot of the books about happiness just could not register with me. I couldn't understand what was wrong with the machine (i.e., humans).

Remember, the assumption is you were born happy. And then something broke; something in this machine became unhappy as I started to engage more and more in modern life.

So I tried to find an equation that describes happiness. And the equation was much simpler than what I thought I would end up finding. I listed down every moment in my life where I felt happy, and I tried to find the trend line. And the trend line was this: every time in my life I felt happy was a moment where life seemed to have been giving me my expectations and wishes and hopes of how life should behave.

I know it sounds silly, but it's almost like a six-year-old. You go to Daddy, and you say, "Daddy, I want a new toy," and if Daddy gives you the new toy, you're happy, if Daddy doesn't have the money or the toy is out of stock, or you've been misbehaving for the last six months, and you really shouldn't get the toy, you feel unhappy.

You don't consider why the toy is not given to you, but you feel unhappy, and that's how we start to interact with life. You can put that in a simple equation: your happiness is equal to or greater than the difference between the events of your life and your hopes and expectations of how life should behave.

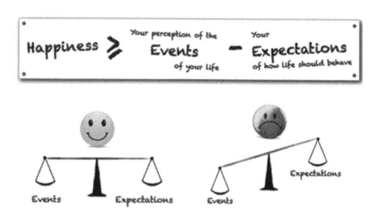

SOURCE: Mo Gawdat, *Solve for Happy* (London: Pan Macmillan, 2019), 26.

Every minute of your day, you're looking around you at tiny things and big things. You're looking at a word that your boyfriend/girlfriend told you, a financial situation you're facing, or a rude driver who made a noise next to you. And every one of those, you're taking them through the happiness equation saying, this event meets my expectations, this event doesn't meet my expectations.

If it meets your expectations, the equation is positive, and you're happy. If it misses your expectations, the equation is negative, and you feel unhappy.

Interestingly, although the equation is correct, we don't always solve it right, and the reason is the factors that we put into that equation are not *really* what's happening in life; it's what we *think* is happening in life.

And these are different.

If you manage to see the difference between them, and you really manage to dive in and see life for what it is, most of your time, your equation will be solved positively.

Thoughts Cause Unhappiness, Not Events

Mo: One of the exercises we do is I say, "Hey, can you please take twenty seconds to think about something that made you unhappy, something in the last week that happened that made you unhappy." And you know what happens? Without fail, everyone in the room will close their eyes and within twenty seconds, [clicks his fingers] unhappiness on demand!

You can easily bring up a thought in your head that makes you unhappy.

But when you manage to get that thought up there and torture yourself, nothing in the real world changes. Right?

So, the second before you brought that thought up was a certain condition of the world, you brought the thought up and started to feel unhappy, and then when you stop thinking about it, you're going to feel happy again. And no impact happens on the real world; no event causes the unhappiness.

It's the thought that causes the unhappiness.

Life has no power over you unless you grant it that power through thinking about it.

And think about it this way: you must have a few friends who are always unhappy, right? What happens is if it's snowing, it's too cold. If it's raining, it's too wet. If it's sunshine, it's too hot.

The event is irrelevant.

Those people look at every possible event in life and find what's wrong with it, not what's right with it. Now, okay, we've learned to go through the modern world and be critical, it's good that you sometimes are analytical, and you see the reality of the world, it's good for you to be successful, but ask yourself this: What does this thought do for you? Does it make your life any better in any way? Does it make people around you who love you happier? Does it make the weather change? When you start to complain about it for hours, will it stop snowing?

It won't.

So, how smart is that? How smart is it that we stay up here [pointing to his head] torturing ourselves with no effect on the real world?

Is It True?

Mo: When you start feeling unhappy, the first thing you should do is trace it back to the thought that generated it. And I say the thought, not the event.

So, the event is "the Uber driver didn't smile." That's the fact of the event.

The thought might be something like, *I was disrespected.*

It's a very different framing of the event than the actual event. If you want to describe the event in very dry words: "Two minutes into my ride, the Uber driver was still not smiling, or he spoke in a loud voice." This is the dry fact.

Now that you know the thought, ask yourself the most important question: Is it true?

Is it true that I was disrespected? Is it true that the Uber driver is supposed to smile? Is it true that this deserves the current unhappiness that I am going through?

If it's true, you ask yourself: can I do something about it?

Can I ping the Uber driver and say, "Don't do that again." Can I maybe rate him three stars? If there is something you can do about it, do it. And when you do it, you're moving the thought from your incessant side of your brain, which causes you unhappiness, to your insightful side of your brain, which is problem-solving and engaging in the real world, where you don't feel unhappy.

If there is nothing you can do about it, can you accept it?

Our Subconscious Brain Can't Process Negatives

Duncan: Our subconscious brain can't process negatives. What does that mean?

Mo: I don't know if you remember, but imagine the time when you were a child, playing with your toes, observing the ceiling.

The only building blocks of knowledge you had were your sensory observations.

So, you could construct knowledge of the world just by observing; you did not have to turn them into words. And then, we start to learn how to use words, and when we use words, they take over as the single building block that we can use to establish knowledge.

So, most of us don't go back and access the subconscious experiences that much. We turn them into words, and we store them as words.

The difference between those two forms of thought is that I can say your T-shirt is not black. *Not black* is something you can describe with language. And if you say, "Not black," my conscious brain can understand that and make a picture of several colors that are not black.

But in the subconscious brain, there is no use of the word 'not.'

So, there is no way I can communicate the word 'not' in the subconscious. So, if I say your T-shirt is not black, the only thing that my subconscious brain understands is 'black."

And this is why when they talk about manifesting the realities of your life, for example, you cannot tell yourself, "I want a life where I don't have this boss," because when you think about, "I don't have this boss…."

Duncan: The picture of the boss pops into your head.

Mo: All that your subconscious brain is seeing is the boss. Boss! Boss! Boss! You're inviting that picture into your observation, into your consciousness.

You have to behave like a child that does not have the word 'not,' who does not negate a concept.

You have to think of the positive concepts to find happiness.

Note: *Although well-intentioned, when we set goals like:*

"I want to stop smoking."

"I want to get out of debt."

"I want to overcome depression."

"I'm going to beat cancer."

What our subconscious registers is: smoking, debt, depression, cancer.

So, to reiterate what Mo said above, make sure you always focus on the picture you want.

For example: health, financial abundance, joy.

Life as a Video Game

Mo: To me, a fulfilled life is to have lived up to the true potential that I had in life.

I think of life more like a video game. I try to go through life in a way that I know life is bound to throw problems at me, I know that the game is going to be tough sometimes, and my fulfillment is not to live a relaxed life; my fulfillment is to engage in the hard parts of the game and learn.

Not to finish the level – who wants to finish the level? You want to enjoy the game. To enjoy the game, you need to learn and engage, accept the challenges, and be the best gamer you can be.

PETER DOCKER

Former Royal Air Force senior officer, former international negotiator for the U.K. Government, co-author of *Find Your Why: A Practical Guide for Discovering Purpose for You and Your Team.*

The narratives we construct in our heads affect our reality. A clear, unequivocal decision is potent. My conversation with Peter was coming to an end when he told me the story below.

Create Your Possibility

Peter: I've got a son Patrick, twenty-three years old, and he's got a friend called Dylan. A couple of years ago, Dylan was riding his motorbike late at night, back from a job that he had then. We live out in the countryside, and there are no streetlights, it's very dark, and the roads are narrow lanes. Unfortunately, on that particular night, a car was coming the other way, a Subaru Impreza, doing a hundred miles an hour, driven by a guy who'd been drinking and he didn't see Dylan, and he hit him.

A car against a young lad on a motorbike. Not much contest. Dylan was thrown over fifty meters, his arms were broken, his back was broken, massive internal injuries, his head was almost severed, but he was still just about alive.

Fortunately, that night, there was an air ambulance in the air. Where the accident had occurred, it was outside of their area, and they were heading back, and they heard the call and said, "Should we go?" and decided they'd go. The paramedics got off the aircraft and managed to stabilize Dylan, one of them was holding his head on. They got him to the hospital, the John Radcliffe in Oxford, and the surgeons did their miracles and managed to save his life.

Some months later, I was driving to our little office, and I went through the village where Dylan lives, and I saw him there. He was in a wheelchair with his mum pushing him around to get some fresh air. I thought *It's Dylan! I've got to go and speak to Dylan.* So, I parked the car, put the brake on, rushed over to him, and said, "Dylan, fantastic to see you! How's it going?"

And he turned to me in his wheelchair, and he said, his voice was thin because the accident had cut through his vocal cords, "Well, it's been tough, I've had many operations, I've just had another one last week where they've taken some nerves from my leg and put them in my arm. Hopefully, I'll get the use of this arm again."

And then he looked up at me, and he said, "In six months, I'm doing a half marathon. Would you sponsor me?"

And I looked at this broken kid, twenty-one years old, in this wheelchair.

Had he any experience at all of walking, let alone running, since his accident?

No.

Was there any doubt in his face when he told me he would run this marathon?

None whatsoever.

Were his words complicated?

No, they weren't; they were very, very simple.

Did I have any doubt of his commitment?

None whatsoever.

I said, "Of course, I'll sponsor you."

At that very moment, Dylan created his possibility.

He inspired others who came along: the doctors, the nurses, the physios, his friends like my son Patrick, to help support him.

And it was a case of, "Right, well, he's signed up!"

"This is happening! Best we get him there!"

Duncan: Incredible.

Peter: Some months later, I was in Dubai giving a talk, and I mentioned Dylan, told the story, and it was a great pleasure as I was able to look at my watch and I said, "Right now, Dylan is running that half marathon."

"All negativity is caused by an accumulation of psychological time and denial of the present.

Unease, anxiety, tension, stress, worry – all forms of fear – are caused by too much future, and not enough presence.

Guilt, regret, resentment, grievances, sadness, bitterness, and all forms of non-forgiveness are caused by too much past, and not enough presence."

ECKHART TOLLE

BRUCE LIPTON, PHD

Cell biologist whose pioneering research presaged
the field of epigenetics (the study of how
environment and perception control one's genes),
bestselling author of *The Biology of Belief*.

*How powerful are we? Can our thoughts change our
biology? Who's in charge, our genes or our beliefs? I had
a lot of unanswered questions, so I called up Dr. Bruce
Lipton.*

The Brain Is the Chemist

Bruce: About forty years ago, I was cloning stem cells. Stem cells
are embryonic cells; they could become anything.

So I have a culture dish; I put one stem cell in it, just one. But
it divides every ten hours, so first there's one cell, then there's
two, then there's four, then there's eight, sixteen, it's doubling
every ten hours. I've got about fifty thousand cells in the Petri
dish at the end of a week.

They all came from one parent. There are fifty thousand genetically identical cells; that's what cloning is. Now, here's where
the experiment shifted my whole career.

I took the cells in the big dish and broke them up into three
smaller Petri dishes.

Three dishes. Genetically identical cells.

To grow cells, you have to grow them in an environment.

What the hell is an environment? What the cells live in.

What is it? Culture medium.

What is a culture medium? That's my laboratory version of blood. In other words, if I grow mouse cells, I look at the composition of mouse blood because that's what the cells normally live in; I make a synthetic version, I call it 'mouse culture medium.'

If I grow human cells, I look at the composition of human blood and create a synthetic version called 'human culture medium,' and I grow cells in it.

Here's the point. Three dishes, genetically identical cells in each dish, but I changed the chemistry of the culture medium a little bit.

And in one dish, the cells form muscle.

In a second dish with slightly different chemistry, a little bit different, the cells form bone.

In the third dish, genetically identical cells but different culture medium, the cells form fat cells.

Okay, one dish muscle, one dish bone, one dish fat cells.

What controls the fate of the cells? They were all genetically identical. So, the first thing is, I can't say, "The genes caused it" – they all had the same genes.

It was the environment!

What's the environment? Culture medium.

Yeah, but what is the culture medium? The equivalent of blood.

Bottom line, the composition of the culture medium – the environment – controls the genetics of the cell.

Now here's the point. Okay, are you excited, Duncan?

Duncan: I'm ready. I'm excited.

Bruce: When you look in the mirror and see yourself, that handsome Duncan looking back – "Hey, I'm Duncan." – you see one organism, but that's a misperception because you are fifty trillion cells.

The cells are the living organism.

You, Duncan, Bruce, whatever, is a name for a community of fifty trillion cells.

Here comes the simple understanding of life now.

We are skin-covered Petri dishes.

We've got fifty trillion cells under the skin.

And you have a culture medium? Yeah, blood!

The chemical composition of the culture medium controls the fate of the cells.

Wait, the chemical composition of my blood is controlling my cells? Yeah.

What controls the chemical composition of your blood?

The brain!

The brain is the chemist.

The mind has pictures. It could be a good picture, could be a bad picture. It has a picture.

What does the brain do? It translates the picture into the chemistry that matches the picture.

So, if I have a picture of love in my brain, my brain takes that picture and converts it into chemistry that includes dopamine – pleasure.

Yeah, being in love, I get pleasure. Where did that come from? Dopamine in the blood gave me pleasure.

What else? Oxytocin.

What's that for? Bonding. Bond to the one that's giving you pleasure. So, my brain is releasing pleasure – dopamine; oxytocin for bonding. It releases growth hormones.

Why? Because it makes you healthy to be in love, and that's why "Ooo, look, they're so in love, you can see how they glow!"

The glow = growth hormone added to your culture medium from your brain.

The brain takes a picture and turns it into the chemistry that matches the picture.

Picture of love = chemistry of health and happiness.

Oh, wait, wait, the same person opens their eyes and sees something that scares them.

You're not releasing dopamine and oxytocin anymore. Now the brain releases stress hormones and inflammatory agents, which have a different effect on the body. They close you down. They get you ready for protection.

So, my body's response was not controlled by genes.

It was controlled by chemistry.

Yeah, but the chemistry is what?

A matching of a thought!

Placebo Effect, Nocebo Effect

Duncan: It can work as a self-fulfilling prophecy, whether our thoughts are empowering or disempowering?

Bruce: Right, and it's a manifestation of our thoughts that becomes the important part. People have understood one aspect of this for a long time but ignored its meaning; it's called *the placebo effect*.

What is the placebo effect? You believe you're going to get well, and the belief healed you, not the pill. Ahh, that's cool, that was a positive belief about healing, and I had a positive effect.

Now here's the killer: what about a negative belief?

It's *equally* powerful to a positive belief, but a negative belief will take you toward disease and death.

We never talk about the negative side. The negative side is called *nocebo*.

And what it means is this: a negative belief will manifest, except when it manifests, it's antagonistic to your welfare, your health, and your life.

So, what's the point?

Whether they're positive or negative, your beliefs are manifesting. Your beliefs are manifesting your life.

You are responsible for your beliefs.

If you have negative beliefs and walk around the world and go, "Oh yeah, geez, I knew that wasn't going to work, and it *didn't*," and "I thought I'd get sick, and I *did!*"

And it's like you don't realize the source was in here [pointing to his head].

Here's the word, Duncan, don't cringe. *Responsibility.* Responsibility.

Duncan: Responsibility, ouch.

Bruce: People don't want to hear that because we've been programmed not to be responsible: "Oh, your life is controlled by genes," "Oh, bacteria viruses are running your life, and you're a wimp, and you're vulnerable, and you're frail."

That's a bunch of B.S.

B.S. means Belief System. That's a bunch of B.S.!

The fact is this: you are so powerful.

You can walk across hot coals!

But you better realize it was a consciousness that got you across the hot coals. If you're in the middle of that walk across the hot coals and have a doubt, for a fraction of a second, just a doubt – *can I do this?* BOOM! You just got burned.

What Can the Mind Do? Testify!

Bruce: Our belief system is, "My biology is out of control and causing all these problems."

No, no. Your mind is out of control. The biology is just conforming to what your mind is.

To show you how effective and powerful the mind is, you can hypnotize somebody and say, "I have here a burning cigarette, and I'm going to touch your arm with a burning cigarette." And you take your finger and touch their arm while they're in hypnosis. Within a minute or two, that individual can express a blister, a whole blister from a burn.

So, where did the blister come from – I touched them with a finger!

No, the mind was creating reality. If the mind saw it got burned, it will manifest a blister whether it got burned or not because the mind is manifesting reality. It saw the burn.

Duncan: Really?

Bruce: Yeah. And why is this relevant?

Every aspect of our life is like that. We are self-sabotaging ourselves.

We look at our lives, like, "My failures in life are because the universe is against me." No, it never was that way. Our failures are in life because our programming is against us.

In the south in the U.S., we have fundamentalist religious people, Baptist Fundamentalists. They work themselves into a state of religious ecstasy where they start speaking in 'tongues' and act like weird, crazy people.

But here's the interesting part: these people do something called *testify*.

Testify – what is that?

You do something that no person in their right mind would ever do because it's so dangerous, but you do it because you know God will protect you – that's what testify is.

Some of them are called snake handlers, and they handle these very poisonous things like rattlesnakes, and they handle them, and the snakes bite them, and they don't have any adverse effects by it.

What do you mean, they got bitten by a snake?

No, their belief in God, their belief in *they're safe*, that's what it is, they attribute it to God – really, it's just they're so sure they're safe – that even being bitten by a rattlesnake doesn't produce the harmful effect.

Okay, those are the minor players. Let me give you the one that I wanted to tell you about. Some drink strychnine poison in toxic doses because they believe God will protect them.

They drink the strychnine poison and have no harmful effects. And the point is, it's because of a belief.

If you drink strychnine poison, you're sure as hell going to have a problem. Then how come they don't? They're not genetically different.

Their mind is so sure that God protects them.

It's the same as walking across hot coals; you don't burn yourself, but the moment you have doubt – your mind is no longer holding that truth – is the moment you could get burned instantly at that point.

Taking a poison is like walking across hot coals but in a way. The poison goes in the system comes out of the system without being taken up by the system. But that's part of the brain.

So, the reality is, what can the mind do?

You can drink strychnine poison and not get sick. That's a damn good start for how powerful it is.

I Think I'm Going to Die Now

Bruce: "Ohh, my father died when he was fifty-one, my grand-father died when he was forty-seven. Jeez, I'm fifty years old, I think I'm going to die now" because that's the belief system.

Or "My mother got cancer, my grandmother had cancer, so I'm going to get cancer."

These are beliefs. If you believe that, you don't need to have a cancer gene. I can make cancer just by having a belief of cancer.

So, the whole message is we've been waiting for people "out there" to make the change. And the answer is, it's not coming from out there.

If you don't change what's going on in here first [pointing to his head], then that world out there will stay just the way it is.

A LIFE TOTALLY ENGAGED IN DOING

MO GAWDAT

"We wake up every morning and rush through a life that is totally engaged in doing. This fast-paced, immersive lifestyle is the opposite of our default nature as humans. It's like living underwater while wearing heavy shoes. Everything around you is hazy, unfamiliar, and heavy. It's hard to move or function naturally. You feel fatigued as you push against the viscosity of the water. You feel the pressure of the depth and the lack of oxygen to breathe. Your eyes burn with the salty water, but you keep trying to find your way, totally exhausted and performing below your best. As harsh as this definition sounds, it's very close to how we go through life while being totally unaware."[8]

CARL HONORÉ

"The godfather of the Slow Movement,"
TED Talker, bestselling author of *In Praise of Slow:
How a Worldwide Movement is Challenging
the Cult of Speed.*

*I first came across Carl after watching his TED talk
'In Praise of Slowness.' He speaks about our roadrunner
culture and the constant hurry of modern life. One day
Carl was scanning an article of time-saving tips for busy
people. The article mentioned a series of one-minute
bedtime stories. He saw the title Snow White in 60
Seconds and thought hallelujah, a way to speed up
bedtime! However, his subsequent thought was very
different. Had his life come to this? Was he going to
shortchange his son with a soundbite at the end of the
day? Did he want to rush through life rather than savor
it? Something had to change.*

How to Take a Vacation Without Checking Emails

Carl: Another example I came across recently which tickled me
was an entrepreneur. I met him on a plane, and we were talking
about the whole problem of defending your vacation from all
the intrusions: the electronic intrusions that come from the
workplace, friends too, social media, but mainly the workplace,
especially in the United States where people tend to take shorter

vacations and they're always getting emails from the office, and they can never get away fully. And this high-flying entrepreneur, very busy, very successful, he said to me, he hadn't had a vacation in years without checking his email several times a day and being distracted.

Then he realized at one point that most of the emails could wait, and so he decided to draw a line in the sand. And the way he did it was he went on a vacation for three or four days, and before going, he put out an automatic reply on his emails, and it said:

Thank you for your email.

I'm away for three days to recharge my batteries. I'm not looking at email.

The reason: to make myself a better version, I will be able to work better, and I'll serve you better when I return.

So, please wait till I get back.

But if this is an irresistibly urgent request that you have, please resend your email to the following address:

RuinMyVacation@gmail.com

Duncan: Haha.

Carl: Haha, and I thought that's inspired, and I said, "Well, that's obviously very amusing. What happened? How did it play out?"

And he said, "Nobody ever wrote to me, and I've carried on doing it. No one's ever written to me on vacation, and I've never missed a job. I've never fallen off on a deadline, the world has never ended while I've been away, and actually, I've heard that some of the people I know in my network started doing something similar."

And I think the fact that he's using humor is also worth re-membering because people often think of slow as being boring, un-fun, lacking in pleasure, and just dull.

Whereas I think the opposite is true, that by slowing down, living fully, enjoying things to the maximum, you're on fire, you're alive, and you see the funny side of things.

Get More Done by Working Less

Duncan: The idea that you can get more done by working less is exciting, but how is that possible? A part of our brain is like, "No, bullshit," but there's science backing this up now, isn't there?

Carl Honoré: There is, there's plenty of science, and the part of our brain that says, "No, bullshit," is the part of our brain that's still thinking about work in terms of the Victorian industrial era. Largely, you turn up at a factory; the harder you work, the more widgets you got through down the line, and the more productive you were.

That's not the way most of us work nowadays.

Most of what we deliver to our employers or ourselves if we're self-employed comes through much more wooly forms of work. So it's making connections socially, creative thinking, and stuff that's very hard to package up and accelerate.

So, when you talk about the benefits of slowing down at the workplace and how you can get more done with less, what we mean is that there are times to shift gears into a slower, more relaxed, more unhurried state. When you do that, the science shows clearly that the brain moves into a richer, more nuanced, more creative mode of thought. Psychologists call that *slow thinking*.

And I think anyone who does any creative work knows that you need moments of silence, moments where you're not distracted by your phone, and several other tasks on your list.

You need to slow down.

And I think that there's a misleading idea in the workplace nowadays, which is that more is more, and I think more and more if I'm not using that word too often in the same sentence, people realize that that's just folly.

Actually, by changing gears, by having moments of slowness, you come back to the faster moments more productive, getting things done more quickly, and that brings me to what I always call the delicious *paradox of slow*.

By slowing down, not only do you get better results, but you often get them faster.

You have to slow down to speed up life is another way of thinking about it.

A little while ago, the *Economist* magazine did an extensive survey looking at the speed and pressures of the modern workplace. They concluded that some things are getting faster, principally information technology. But other things are not getting quicker, and in fact, you need to keep a slower beat going at the same time as the beat accelerates in other ways in the workplace.

And the final paragraph of that survey from the *Economist* was a perfect, very *Economist*, pithy summation of the slow philosophy that I've been espousing for years now. It said simply:

"Forget frantic acceleration; mastering the clock of business means choosing when to be fast and when to be slow."

And there it is, in very few words, in a nutshell.

And that's the *Economist* magazine; it's not *Buddhist Monthly*, it's not *Acupuncture Weekly*, it's the in-house bible of the go-getters, the entrepreneurs, the fast movers, the move-fast-and-break-things crowd. That's the magazine they will turn to, to work out how to make sense of the world, and that magazine is saying the same thing that I'm saying, and anyone else who embraces this slow revolution is saying, which is that slow has a role to play in the twenty-first century.

A big role!

ROKO BELIC

Academy Award-nominated filmmaker. Writer, director, and co-producer of *Happy*.

Tom Shadyac (the director of Ace Ventura, Bruce Almighty, and The Nutty Professor) was reading an article in the New York Times one morning. It described how America was a very wealthy country, but not a happy one. Tom was making millions of dollars on every film, and he knew the millions were not making him happy. The question he wanted to know was, what does work? He called up Roko and asked him whether he'd be willing to make a documentary film exploring this question. The result was the film Happy.

Happiness Intervention

Roko: A happiness intervention, meaning, how do I become happier right now, with a small activity?

If you express your appreciation to somebody, it could be your first-grade teacher, it could be a neighbor that you used to live next to twenty years ago, but just by expressing that appreciation, whether it's in an email or writing a letter or making a phone call, the expression of it actually boosts your happiness not only for minutes, but it could be hours, even days, even *weeks* after you do it.

Isn't that amazing? Even if you don't know if the person ever heard the message, writing the damn letter, just writing it, can boost your happiness significantly for up to days and weeks later.

Every Happy Person Has This in Common

Roko: When I asked the leading researcher, "What's the key to happiness?"

He said, "Well, it's different for different people, but…"

Every happy person he's ever studied for thirty-five years, who's very happy, has strong relationships.

It doesn't mean that those people love everybody or they're the life of the party, they don't have to be a jokester, but it means that they love somebody and somebody loves them.

It's sort of that simple.

DAVID RAICHLEN, PHD

Professor of Human and Evolutionary Biology at USC, former postdoctoral fellow at Harvard University, studies how exercise affected the trajectory of human evolution.

I was learning a lot about the way our mind affects our body. But what about the reverse: how does the way we move our body affect our mind and our mental health? I began tracking down experts to help shed some light on this. First, I wanted to speak with a biologist to determine what evolution had to say.

For Two Million Years, No One Had to Make This Decision

David: We have a drive to save energy. Our bodies don't want to spend energy; it feels good to sit down and relax. There's an evolutionary reason for that. The energy you spend on an activity you can't spend on reproduction.

But our physiology evolved within the context of activity.

For two million years, no one had to make the decision – should I or shouldn't I exercise? You had to!

You don't get to choose not to move your body as a hunter-gatherer, or else you don't eat. So, the decision to exercise was never a part of our evolutionary requirements.

If You Don't Use It, You Lose It

Duncan: "Nothing in biology makes sense except in the light of evolution," according to Theodosius Dobzhansky. Do you believe in that statement?

David: Yes, I think this is one of the most profound concepts we have to work with. It is difficult to understand concepts in health, biology, medicine, etc., without firmly grounding them in evolutionary theory.

We live in the physiology of hunter-gatherers.

Over the last ten thousand years, we've had some changes with agriculture and whatnot, but the way that our physiology works is a function of this highly active hunting and gathering past. When we become inactive, when we become sedentary, there are some real evolutionary reasons why our physiology responds negatively to that behavior.

If you don't need something, your body takes it away.

That's an evolutionary solution to an energy expenditure problem. If you're not using it, shrink it so you're not spending the energy on it.

Same thing with our bones. If you're not stressing them with forces, why maintain a lot of bone mass? Our bodies are smart. Save energy! Reduce bone mass!

But down the line, that creates some problems. Our physiology evolved to be active, and if we don't use our bodies that way, we lose that physiological capacity.

It's the same thing with your brain.

Our brains evolved within the context of physical activity. And our brains respond to physical activity in a certain way.

And if you don't get your body moving, your brain reacts negatively.

That's true of mental health.

Our brains evolved in the context of neurotransmitter activity that occurred during exercise, and so, our brains require that activity.

WHY DO WE HAVE BRAINS?

DANIEL WOLPERT, PHD, FRS

"Why do we and other animals have brains? Not all species on our planet have brains, so if we want to know what the brain is for, let's think about why we evolved one.

"Now, you may reason that we have one to perceive the world or to think, and that's completely wrong. If you think about this question for any length of time, it's blindingly obvious why we have a brain. We have a brain for one reason and one reason only, and that's to produce adaptable and complex movements. There is no other reason to have a brain. Think about it; movement is the only way you have of affecting the world around you. That's not quite true, there's one other way, and that's through sweating, but apart from that, everything else goes through contractions of muscle.

"So, think about communication: speech, gestures, writing, sign language; they're all mediated through contractions of your muscles. So, it's really important to remember that sensory memory and cognitive processors are all important, but they're only important to either drive or suppress future movements.

There can be no evolutionary advantage to laying down memories of childhood or perceiving the color of a rose if it doesn't affect the way you're going to move later in life.

"For those who don't believe this argument, we have trees and grass on our planet without the brain, but the clinching evidence is this animal...the humble sea squirt. Rudimentary animal; has a nervous system, swims around in the ocean in its juvenile life, and at some point in its life, it implants on a rock, and the first thing it does when implanting on that rock, which it never leaves, is to digest its own brain and nervous system for food. So, once you don't need to move, you don't need the luxury of that brain."[9]

JOHN RATEY, MD

Neuropsychiatrist, Massachusetts Psychiatric Society's Outstanding Psychiatrist of the Year, bestselling author of *Spark: The Revolutionary New Science of Exercise and the Brain.*

One name kept on coming up again and again. Research, book suggestions, and personal recommendations led me to the same man: Dr. John Ratey. There is no question that exercise is vital for our physical health, but is this a sideshow to what it can do for our mental health?

We've Known This for 2,400 Years

Duncan: We've known about the effect of exercise on our mood since Hippocrates – that was his treatment for depression in 300/400 BC. The American Psychiatric Association in 2010 finally approved exercise as a viable treatment for depression; if we've known about this for two thousand four hundred years, why did it take so long?

John: It was hard to get double-blind placebo-controlled studies that people would believe. We had them, but it took one psychiatrist who stood in both camps – the camps of psychopharmacology and exercise – Dr. Madhukar Trivedi from Texas. He was a world expert in psychopharmacology, which was leading the way in the American Psychiatric Association for the longest time. He said, hey, I'm doing both, these both work; what are we doing not putting it in there? But the evidence was accumulating overwhelmingly. And great studies, coming out of Duke University, coming out of the University of Texas, not just in the U.S. but worldwide. People were getting proof that exercise was a good way to unlock the moods, make it better, and prevent depression from coming on.

It shows you, I think, medicine in general; I go back to Niels Bohrs' quote, who said, "Old scientists don't change their mind, they just die."

Duncan: Haha.

John: Haha, it's hard for people who have spent their lifetime proving in one area, in one silo, to go outside that, and I think that's a reason why it takes so long for any field to change.

Exercise Is Miracle-Gro for the Brain

Duncan: You refer to exercise as "Miracle-Gro for the Brain," i.e., brain fertilizer. Why is that? I know it ties into this thing called BDNF?

John: Yes. BDNF – that's one thing people should go away sort of saying, "I want more BDNF," "I need more BDNF!"

Why?

Well, BDNF, we discovered in the early eighties. Its proper name is *brain-derived neurotrophic factor.*

It's what I call evolution's gift to us. It's a protein that gets released when our brain cells fire. And the beauty of it is it gets released, and then it helps manage the brain, it helps the brain cells it's released from, and the cells around it grow.

There are a lot of growth factors, but this is the major, the mother of all growth factors.

When we release it, it sends a signal back to the brain cell that released it to turn on the genetic machinery and then the protein-building machinery in our brain to make more of it.

So, it's a self-generating cycle that if we're firing our brain cells, we will make more of this stuff, and then when we make more of this stuff, we're going to have a healthy, healthy brain.

And one thing we know is that along with all these other great things like dopamine and norepinephrine and serotonin and all that's released when we fire our brain cells, we release this BDNF, and it presents the perfect soup for our brain cells to grow.

In 2003, Nobel Prizes were given to the guys who found and showed that the way we learn anything is for our brain cells to grow.

So, we want to keep our brain cells growing because if we don't, they start eroding.

"What virtually no one recognizes…is that inactivity is killing our brains."

John Ratey, MD

The Naperville Experiment

Note: *In the 1990s, a Naperville school district in Illinois implemented a physical education program designed to improve the student's fitness levels, rather than just their sporting ability.*

There were eighteen fitness options for the kids to choose from, from basketball to rock climbing, and they'd wear heart monitors to track their improvements.

Not only did this affect their bodies, but it affected their minds.

John: In 1999, ninety-seven percent of the kids took the TIMSS test, the international science, and math test to evaluate all countries every three years. The U.S. takes it, and we're in the mid-teens somewhere in science and math compared to all the other countries. Schools in Asia and Finland are always in the top five. But you could lobby to take it as a country, and Naperville took it as a country.

Duncan: That was interesting. Not as a school in America; they put themselves forward as a country, just their school district.

John: Yes, to compare to other countries. And they came in number one in the world in science and number six in math.

This was like, "What?"

Exercising didn't take away from their studies. Nineteen thousand kids in their school district, among the fittest kids in the world, and the smartest! So, that got me on an airplane to Naperville to see what was going on, and I was just amazed.

Ministry of Loneliness

John: In the U.K., for instance, in 2002-2003, the House of Commons said, okay, we know that people who are depressed or anxious and prisoners of their house need to get out and exercise, so they passed a bill of some sort saying every community will have a center that will provide mentors or companions to get people who are depressed out walking.

Of course, there was no money to follow that, it never got in place, but there was an appreciation that this is a way we need to work on things.

Three years ago, when I was over talking in the U.K., they had just created a Ministry of Loneliness.

Duncan: I did not know that.

John: No, most people don't know about it, don't hear about it, but that's a huge problem.

Not just for the aging but for a large part of the population who are wedded to their cellphones.

Big Changes in Medicine

John: The biggest tsunami coming is the aging issue and losing our brains. Everybody has stories of somebody they know and love who has lost their minds as they age, cognitive decline, and dementia, everybody, it's all over. And so, a huge change has been looking at what we need to do to prevent that, and the big move today is to decrease inflammation, neural inflammation, in the brain. And that happens to be important for all the psychiatric issues, depression, anxiety, but certainly for aging the brain. And the number one recommendation is exercising.

Another change is that we have a big movement here called Exercise is Medicine for the Brain – and that's amongst medical professionals.

It's people saying, "Yes, we have *this* and *that* drug with *this* and *that* drug because the drug companies have the money and they have Madison Avenue." [P.R. and advertising]

But what they are coming to, even in cancer therapy, is that you might do your anti-cancer treatment with drugs and radiation and surgery but the number one recommendation after that is to stay moving! Get moving!

GRAHAM HANCOCK

Researcher, editor of *The Divine Spark: Psychedelics, Consciousness and the Birth of Civilization*, bestselling author of *Fingerprints of the Gods*.

We have an interesting relationship with medicines. Some we will consume daily. Others we will outlaw and lock people up associated with them. But if some can help people, is this approach doing more harm than good? I wanted to learn more about psychedelics and how they are being used to heal. I first spoke with Graham Hancock and then with Dennis McKenna, PhD.

Therapeutic Uses of Psychedelic Medicines

Graham: More cross-cultural research needs to be done on the Amazonian plant medicine *ayahuasca*. Certain aspects of the ayahuasca experience crop up again and again all over the world, regardless of the setting. Whether it's a big city or the middle of a jungle, whether the people had compared notes or not, whether or not they knew anything about ayahuasca before they drank it, there are these astonishing transpersonal connections. As though all of us are peering into the same, usually invisible, parallel realm. This is what's remarkable about ayahuasca, and it's why I feel that much more detailed research needs to be done.

Duncan: One example of where it's being used to heal is Takiwasi clinic in Peru.

Graham: Takiwasi clinic in Peru. They are getting drug addicts, people addicted to really harmful drugs like heroin and cocaine, getting them off their addictions to those hard drugs with ayahuasca.

A month of ayahuasca sessions will produce a revelation that results in well over fifty percent of the subjects completely giving up their hard drug habit, breaking their addiction, no withdrawal symptoms, and no return. No return to drug addiction.

Astonishing results, yet Dr. Gabor Maté was getting the same results in Canada, but he was stopped; he was banned by the Canadian authorities on the grounds that ayahuasca is a drug, but this is an extraordinary new avenue for ending drug addiction.

Ayahuasca is primarily about healing, that's what it's always been about in the Amazon jungle, and that's the role it plays today. So again, we have to abandon; we have to take off these ideological blinkers and look at things as they are.

Duncan: If it can tick all the right boxes in the medical arena, does that open the door to its exploration in other areas?

Graham: Yes, absolutely, this is the beginning of the change. In the last decade, we have witnessed a resurgence of the study of the therapeutic outcomes of psychedelics, and they have been enormously helpful to people suffering from a range of conditions, from cluster headaches to anxiety about death in terminal cancer patients.

Psilocybin has been clinically shown to: radically reduce that anxiety, give the patient the sense that life doesn't end with physical death, that we aren't just physical creatures, that we are this mysterious consciousness incarnated in a physical form, and when the physical form comes to an end, why, that's no more serious than discarding an old suit. The consciousness continues.

This is the revelation of psychedelics.

Now, is the revelation real?

That's another question. We need to do the research to find that out.

But does the revelation itself have therapeutic effects?

Yes! Absolutely. That has been demonstrated already.

So, scientists are beginning, and it's risky for them because anybody who speaks positively about psychedelics in our society is immediately subjected to a massive ideological attack.

DENNIS McKENNA, PHD

Ethnopharmacologist, founding board member
of the Heffter Research Institute, a non-profit
organization dedicated to investigating therapeutic
uses of psychedelic medicines.

Psychedelics Teach You a Lot of Things

Dennis: I think it's critical to be able to step out of your reference frame temporarily. We get so wound up in ourselves, and we tend to believe we are important, particularly in the West. This attitude has poisoned Western culture.

Psychedelics teach you; they teach you a lot of things.

They teach you, number one, that you don't know so much; they make you aware of the limitations of our knowledge, how little we know.

And they teach you about this connection to everything, every other being, and everything in the universe. These habits that we've developed that there are barriers, there are boundaries, that's an illusion. We really are all one. That's a profound appreciation if you can internalize that.

And then the other thing I think it teaches you, the fact that we know so little, encourages humility. Essentially, it discourages arrogance because it shows right into your face how little we know, and that's a good thing.

Alienation Is the Word of Our Times

Dennis: *Alienation* is kind of the key word of our times.

Alienation from ourselves, alienation from each other, and alienation from nature.

CAN MONEY BUY YOU HAPPINESS?

A Harvard Business School study by Michael Norton, Elizabeth Dunn, and Lara Aknin investigated whether money can buy you happiness.

They gave money to strangers ($5 or $20), and they told them to spend it that day. Half were instructed to spend it on themselves; half were told to spend it on others.

The participants who spent it on others reported feeling a lot happier at the end of the day than those who bought stuff for themselves.

The amount of money didn't matter; these findings were consistent regardless of the sum.[10]

"Several similar studies confirm that money can indeed buy you happiness – if you give it away. So does everything you have to give: your smile, your time, attention, knowledge, compliment."

MO GAWDAT

DO YOU ADD VALUE
OR TAKE VALUE?

Are you an asset or a liability? A value adder or taker? Do you make situations, places, people's lives better or worse?

I think it falls into one of two categories, and all day, every day, we have the opportunity to be the former. You're in a supermarket, and you give a genuine smile or a thank you to the checkout person; you're in a cafe, you see something on the floor, and you throw it in the bin.

How can I make this place, this person's life, this situation, just that little bit better?

Because you're reading this book, I'm assuming you're interested in the question: "How can I make my life better?"

Focus on making other people's lives better.

If you want something, focus on giving it.

If you want more friendship in your life, focus on being a better friend.

If you want more people to care about you, focus on caring about others first.

If you're a giver, you don't need to worry about what you can get because people will want to help you, want to look out for you, and want to spend time with you.

However, this advice is not to be misunderstood or confused with being a selfless giver or a martyr where you put everyone's needs and desires ahead of your own until you burn out or become a doormat.

Adam Grant, Wharton professor and author of *Give and Take*, describes the difference between two giving styles.

"There's this…group of givers that I call "otherish." They are concerned about benefitting others, but they also keep their own interests in the rearview mirror. They will look for ways to help others that are either low cost to themselves or even high benefit to themselves, i.e., win-win, as opposed to win-lose. Here's the irony. The selfless givers might be more altruistic, in principle, because they are constantly elevating other people's interests ahead of their own. But my data, and research by lots of others, show that they're actually less generous because they run out of energy, they run out of time, and they lose their resources because they basically don't take enough care of themselves. The "otherish" givers are able to sustain their giving."[11]

STEVEN KOTLER

Two-time Pulitzer Prize-nominated writer, peak performance expert, bestselling author of *The Rise of Superman: Decoding the Science of Ultimate Human Performance.*

Two of my favorite thinkers are Steven Kotler and Peter Diamandis. I love big thinkers and ideas that stretch my understanding of what is possible for individuals and humanity. Steven has spent decades exploring the outer edges of human potential and demonstrating that we are capable of far more than we realize.

Flow States

Duncan: You had a debilitating illness, only about ten percent functional; you had been bedbound for almost three years. How did flow states help bring you back to life?

Steven: Yeah, so it was a radical experience. As you pointed out, I'd been sick for about three years. I had Lyme disease, and the doctors had pulled me off drugs. There was nothing else anybody could do for me, and I was suicidal. I was going to kill myself because I could work forty minutes a day, and the rest of the time, I could lie on the couch and moan. In the middle of the question of when was I going to do it, a friend shows up at my house and demands that we go surfing. It was a ridiculous request; I couldn't walk across a room, forget about going surfing, but she wouldn't leave and wouldn't leave and wouldn't leave and kept badgering me. After three or four hours of this, I was like, *Whatever, I can kill myself tomorrow; let's just go surfing, anything to get her to shut up.*

She took me out to the waves. They had to walk me out to the break – I couldn't walk out there on my own. They gave me a board the size of a Cadillac. A couple of seconds later, a wave came. It was a tiny day, maybe a two-foot little wave, but I spun the board around, paddled a couple of times, and popped up into a different dimension, a dimension I didn't even know existed. My senses were incredibly heightened; time was passing strangely.

And the craziest part was, I felt great. I felt better than normal; I felt amazing, the best I'd felt in years. I felt so good that I caught a couple more waves that day and had these same quasi-mystical experiences.

Afterward, I went home, was disassembled, couldn't move for a couple of weeks, but when I could walk around again, I went back to the ocean. I did it again, had the same crazy quasi-mystical experience, and over the course of six to eight months, when the only thing I was doing differently was surfing and having these strange altered state experiences, I got better. I went from ten percent functionality up to about eighty percent functional.

And so, my first question was, what the hell's going on?

On top of the fact that I was feeling better and surfing should not be a cure for chronic autoimmune conditions, I was having these quasi-mystical experiences in the waves. I'm a science guy – I don't have quasi-mystical experiences ever! I was sure the disease had gotten into my brain, and it was rotting my brain; that's why I was having these experiences.

So it lit up a giant question to figure out what the hell was going on with me. And the first thing I discovered is that these strange states of consciousness that I was getting into had a name: flow states.

They're moments of optimal performance when we feel our best and perform our best; it's those states of total rapt attention and focused absorption where you're so concentrated on what you're doing, on the task at hand, that everything else disappears.

And all aspects of performance, mental and physical, go through the roof.

I also discovered a big neurobiological change happens in the body when we move into these states.

Two important things happen concerning my story.

First, the nervous system gets reset, so all the stress hormones get flushed out of the system as you move into flow, which calms the nervous system down.

An autoimmune condition is a nervous system gone haywire, so calming my nervous system down was a big deal.

The other thing is, there's a bunch of neurochemicals that show up in flow. All of them boost the immune system.

So, the combination is what allowed me to get back to health.

But what I quickly discovered, and the reason we're talking today is that the same state of consciousness that got me from super subpar back to normal was helping normal people go all the way up to Superman.

> **Note**: *The work of Mihaly Csikszentmihalyi, Steven Kotler, and Jamie Wheal, among others, has shown that there are multiple 'flow state triggers' that, when present during an activity, dramatically increase the person's likelihood of getting into flow.*

A few examples are:

- *Challenging yourself and stretching your skills to the utmost*
- *Being completely present on the task at hand*
- *Getting immediate feedback*
- *Having a clear goal*
- *Being in novel and stimulating environments*

DIFFICULT
AND WORTHWHILE

MIHALY CSIKSZENTMIHALYI, PHD

"Contrary to what we usually believe...the best moments in our lives are not the passive, receptive, relaxing times – although such experiences can also be enjoyable, if we have worked hard to attain them. The best moments usually occur when a person's body or mind is stretched to its limits in a voluntary effort to accomplish something difficult and worthwhile... For a child, it could be placing with trembling fingers the last block on a tower she has built, higher than any she has built so far; for a swimmer, it could be trying to beat his own record; for a violinist, mastering an intricate musical passage. For each person, there are thousands of opportunities, challenges to expand ourselves."[12]

TAL BEN-SHAHAR, PHD

Taught two of the largest classes in Harvard University's history, bestselling author of *Happier: Learn the Secrets to Daily Joy and Lasting Fulfillment.*

Happiness researchers often have different definitions of what the term means to them. I don't think of happiness and sadness as being opposites. Happiness, to me, is not about always being in a good mood or feeling positive every second of the day. It is a deeper and richer experience. Pain is not an enemy; sadness is not something to avoid. Instead, they are beautiful, challenging parts of life. You don't have to be upbeat always. If you feel sadness, you're not doing anything wrong. A phrase I often think about is one that Dr. Tal taught me: give yourself 'permission to be human.'

The Benefits of Feeling Pain

Duncan: Medicate our problems away, medicate away every painful emotion we experience. Why is this not the right approach?

Tal: Medication is a complex issue because there are cases, some of which I know intimately, where medication has saved lives, so there is certainly a place for it.

The problem with medication comes when we overprescribe; someone is experiencing a painful emotion – their girlfriend dumps them, or they did poorly on an exam – and they resort to medication. Or the medical doctors prescribe psychiatric medication because the people are feeling down, and that's the wrong thing to do, so we overprescribe, that is the problem.

Why?

Because if you go to a room and there are a hundred people in the room, and you ask them to think back to their most important growth experiences, probably ninety-seven or ninety-eight of them would think about painful experiences – it was when the love of my life, or I thought they were the love of my life, dumped me, or when I didn't get a job that I really, really wanted, or I didn't get into a program that I thought was my calling, that's where I learned the most, that's where I grew the most.

Now, if we medicated away every pain we experienced, we're not going to have these growth experiences.

This is important today; it will be even more important ten years from now because the medication will be a lot more precise. It's not going to have the side effects that it has today. It's going to be a lot more readily available. Then people, whenever they experience painful emotions, they're going to go to it, it's going to be so easy to fix, and I think that's unfortunate.

There's a lot of value in also – not only of course – but *also* experiencing pain, disappointment, sadness, and anxiety.

It's all part of a full and fulfilling life.

Duncan: The happiest people are those who open themselves up to this and allow themselves to feel that full range of emotions.

Tal: Exactly right. The Lebanese poet Kahlil Gibran said that every time we experience suffering, it's like we're digging deep into our container, our emotional container, and that container also holds our pleasurable emotions. So it gets bigger with pain, and we have a larger capacity for joy.

Duncan: An interesting study I saw on one of your videos, after a tragedy, people who break down, cry, share are much more likely to get over that tragedy quicker than the people who say, "Stiff upper lip, I'm going to be strong." Those people struggle for longer.

Tal: Exactly. The people who give themselves what I've come to call the 'permission to be human,' whether it's to talk about, to cry, to go through the emotion and the motion, they're much more likely to experience what psychologists today call 'post-traumatic growth' and to develop as a result.

The Dangers of Losing Face Time

Duncan: One of the number one predictors of well-being and happiness is quality time spent with friends and family. However, in the modern world, this quality time is eroding more and more.

Tal: This is a huge issue, and it's a massive issue in today's culture because we spend less face-to-face time with people.

FB time has taken over BF time.

This is unfortunate. I'm not against Facebook; I recently was contacted by a person I hadn't seen for thirty-three years, who was my best friend when I was eleven years old. Facebook is wonderful in that way, but not if it comes in the way of actual meetings, of getting together, playing together in the sandbox.

For two reasons.

The first reason is that one thousand friends on Facebook are no substitute for that one best friend in terms of happiness levels.

There's a direct correlation between loneliness and the amount of time we spend in front of the screen.

So, some screen is great – but too much screen, not great at all.

We need to be together, go for meals together, and by the way, when we go for meals together, not to be texting all the time during those meals, to *really* be together, to switch off, to disconnect so that we can connect.

So that's one thing. The second thing where it really hurts us and potentially will hurt society in the long term is that levels of empathy are lower due to fewer face-to-face interactions.

We develop empathy, not when we talk on the computers. We develop empathy when we play together, fight together, and are in the same room together.

Lots of Money or Lots of Time?

Duncan: That's what we call *time affluence*?

Tal: Yes, Tim Kasser makes the distinction between material affluence and time affluence.

Material affluence is not a predictor of happiness.

And I'm not talking about people living in poverty; additional money would make them happier because they'd have food on the table and their basic needs met, but extra money doesn't make a difference.

But time affluence is the feeling we have time to spend with people we care about, to play – play's another vital component of happiness – and when we're not constantly chasing our own tails and feeling overwhelmed.

Time affluence is a key determinant of happiness.

HIDE AND SEEK

11:45. Tuesday morning. London.

All of my friends are at work. Most of them work in beautiful offices – they're bankers, insurance brokers, and lawyers. They have big salaries.

I'm also at work. In my left hand, I'm holding onto three dogs. In my right hand, there are two bags of poo. I've just started working as a dog walker for *Precious Pooch*.

I look up and see a girl from school that I used to fancy.

"Duncan!" she says. "Oh my God, it's been years! How have you been?"

"Good," I say. "Yeah, good, really, really good." I try to hide the dog shit. "Ermm, business is going really well, starting to get some good momentum…some good traction, have a few interesting, potential projects in the pipeline…."

Later in the afternoon, I get a phone call from my friend Ryan. He tells me about this cool startup he's working for and explains how I could make some money.

"If you're a U.K. resident and have a good credit rating, you can leverage that," he says.

I'm not sure what the word *leverage* means.

Ryan continues, "My company has a network of people all over the U.K. who use their credit score to order mobile phones. In exchange, my company pays them fifty pounds for every phone they order."

———

I adore my parents. They're so supportive and loving; I feel like I can talk to them about anything. But in some ways, we're very different. If I tell my dad a business idea, his way of showing his love is to brainstorm all the potential problems and pitfalls with that idea.

Sure, this is important to know, but it's the least fun way to start any new project.

When I was in Morocco, I met a carpet maker, and I decided that I would invest my entire student loan on ten carpets, ship them back to London, and resell them for a handsome profit.

I call up my dad.

Ten minutes later, my carpet empire is over before it's even begun.

Six months later, I applied and got accepted into a flu camp. Here, the scientists will inject me with something and see what happens over the next fourteen days. Free food, unlimited movies, and £2,000. No-brainer! Right?

Both my parents get involved this time. They give me an hour lecture, and that's the end of flu camp.

So, this time 'round, I'm not telling them. I'm deciding for myself. I tell Ryan to sign me up. Four phones arrive in the post, two from O2 and two from Vodaphone. I give them to Ryan, and his company transfers me £200.

Easy!

I'm an entrepreneur!

————

Eight months have passed. Every few days, I receive a new bill from O2 or Vodaphone. The numbers are getting bigger every time, so I stop opening them.

Ryan is not answering my calls. The envelopes now have words in big red letters on the outside like 'Final Notice' and 'Urgent.'

Every day, I wake up early to collect the post before my parents see it, and then I hide the letters addressed to me in a drawer in my bedroom.

I find out the police have raided the company; they're charging them with fraud and money laundering. All of their computers have been seized for evidence.

The letters keep arriving; I keep hiding them. The pile is getting bigger and bigger.

My name's added to a private Facebook group, others involved, people from all over the country, sharing details about lawyers and updates of the police investigation.

I leave the group. I don't want anything to do with it. It feels dirty. I feel dirty.

————

"Would you like a cup of tea?" my mum asks.

I burst into tears.

My body is shaking.

I can't stop crying; I can't look at either of them.

I'm staring at the cushion on my lap, covering it in tears.

My mum sits down next to me.

She holds me in her arms.

And she says, "You've been raped, haven't you? It's okay. We love you. It's okay."

I haven't been, and I'm not sure why she thinks that. But there is so much kindness in the room, so much compassion, that it is okay.

I tell them everything.

And for the first time in almost a year, I'm free.

BRUCE MUZIK

Relationship repair expert, more than twenty-five years of coaching experience, TEDx Talk viewed by millions.

I spoke to Bruce when I lived in Sri Lanka, and he was in the Dominican Republic. Ten minutes into our chat, the call cut out. Shit. Had my computer crashed? No, it was okay. I checked the internet connection. Also, okay. Fantastic, it wasn't my fault! About forty minutes later, Bruce reappeared; he was very apologetic. Some construction work was happening nearby, and the entire block lost power. He walked to a nearby town to let me know and apologize. He had nothing to apologize for; I'm thrilled when it's not me who screws up. We rescheduled the interview for the next day. Seconds before the new call began my power plummets. I can either have the lights on or the internet on, not both. I chose the internet. Interviewing in the dark felt seventy percent less professional and a hundred percent creepier. But the conversation was fantastic.

What Are You Not Telling?
What Are You Keeping Secret?

Duncan: Would you say that most of us are hiding secrets to some degree or presenting a version of ourselves to the world that isn't authentically who we are?

Bruce: Yes, it's how evolution has designed us to survive. Let me tell you a little bit of backstory about why this is. When I'm saying everybody's a liar, I don't mean it with any malice in my tone of voice because I'll be the first to raise my hand.

So, what we tend to do as human beings is we lie about the small stuff all the time, and how this came about from an evolutionary perspective is, if you imagine being a caveman on the plains of Africa. And you've got your little tribe, and you're with your group of people. Your tribe was what kept you alive. Nature has wired into us or hardwired into us this fear of being ejected from the tribe because if we were rejected from the tribe and left to fend for ourselves on the plains of Africa, a lion would come within half an hour, eat us, and we'd be done.

So, one of the biggest threats to our survival is being ejected from the tribe, as far as evolution is concerned.

Even if that doesn't necessarily present a risk today in our modern twenty-first century because we can all survive on our own or find a new tribe if we need to, it's still like that.

So, to prevent ourselves from being rejected from the tribe, what we do is we present a mask, our ego if you like, to the world, and sometimes we wear it tight and then sometimes we take it off, and we allow our authentic self to shine through.

And we present our mask to the world as an interface through which we can navigate safely and make sure we never get rejected from the tribe.

So, when somebody says, "Hey, how are you doing, Duncan?" Your initial response is, "I'm doing great! I'm awesome." You're probably not going to say, "I'm really sad" or "I don't know how I'm going to pay the bills at the end of the month, and I'm anxious about that." We don't do that because we're expecting somebody to look at us and go, "Ooh, weirdo," and then we're ejected from the tribe.

So, we lie all the time.

What was that stat from my TED Talk, from the Massachusetts professor?

Duncan: Oh yeah, Robert Feldman, a professor of psychology at the University of Massachusetts. He said that when two people meet for the first time, within the first ten minutes, they each, on average, lie three times.

Bruce: That's eighteen times an hour when we first meet each other; we're presenting some kind of falseness. And that's all good and well except that when we're not able to express ourselves authentically in the world, it numbs us.

It kills our sense of aliveness.

If you imagine we have a hosepipe, and this hosepipe flows energy, it's our aliveness; it's what makes us feel alive. When we're not able to be ourselves, it's like there's a kink in the hosepipe, and part of our energy can't flow. And the thing is, human beings are so good at adapting that we get used to the kink after a while, and we forget what it's like to feel alive, and feeling numb becomes normal, and we forget that there's more.

And so we walk around life presenting this mask – my mask is called Bruce, yours is called Duncan – this mask to the world of who we think we are and never really interacting heart to heart with each other; we're communicating mask to mask with each other.

And an amazing thing happens when you take the mask off and start telling the truth. That's how you take the mask off – you start telling the truth about what's going on for you, minute by minute, moment by moment.

You start to feel alive again.

That kink in your energy hosepipe unkinks itself, energy starts to flow through, aliveness comes back, and the smile on your face comes back, and happiness comes back.

And for me, I think one of the highest leveraged things you can do to get to a fulfilled life is to start telling the truth about what you're experiencing moment by moment.

Now that's one level, Duncan, and feel free to interrupt me.

Duncan: No, I'm just sitting back and listening because this is fascinating.

Bruce: The other level is what happens when you're withholding a big secret. So, if you've got something that you've done, perhaps violated one of your values, or let's say you've had an affair, or maybe you've stolen money or something like that, what happens is energetically that weighs down on you, and that you can handle.

But the secondary impact is that the person with whom you've violated that trust or with whom you're keeping that secret from you can no longer be intimate with them.

And that's fine when it's somebody you don't care about – "Well, I'll go and find another friend."

But when it's a child of yours, or you're married to that person, or it's family, you can't just push those relationships to the side. Let's say you've had an affair and you're not talking about it – and this is something that I went through myself, I was the one who had an affair, cheated on my wife, didn't talk about it, bloated up thirty pounds in a couple of months and became depressed.

If you're withholding something fundamental from somebody you love, there's a massive loss of connection.

And that loss of connection will usually result in feeling like you're depressed, you feel numb, your body perhaps gets ill, you gain weight, your energy drops, you sleep a lot.

And my personal belief is that half of depression, like when clients come to me and tell me they're depressed, the first thing I go through is, I ask them, "What are you not telling? What are you not sharing? What are you keeping secret?"

And when we get to that, and they tell that secret, they're like, "Oh my God, depression's gone." They didn't need pills; they didn't need psychotherapy.

Our body knows how to look after itself when we tell the truth and be ourselves.

I was married for five years, and I was cheating on her for the last three years. I got fat, I was depressed, I was a motivational speaker at the time and standing on stage inspiring people, and I felt like a complete fraud.

So, I went and told the truth, and it was brutal, and at the same time, within a week, I felt more alive than I'd ever felt in my life before.

We both decided together, amicably, to get a divorce, and it was probably the best thing we could have done. A week later, she met the man of her dreams, who she's married to now. And that was thirteen years ago, and I haven't felt depressed since that day. Of course, I've had my ups and downs like all of us do, but I haven't gone to a bout of depression or sadness that lasted forever because I'm no longer suffering.

I was able, to tell the truth about who I am.

And then I went and shared a TED Talk and told three million people that I cheated on my wife and used to be a racist. So, there's pretty much nothing I'm ashamed of anymore, and living in the space of no shame, I'm able to feel completely fulfilled and happy.

I can wake up every day knowing that I like who I am. I'm not hiding who I am. You like me, or you don't, and that's okay.

It's been the most freeing thing I've ever done.

If We Didn't Forgive Each Other, Nothing Would Change

Duncan: The Truth and Reconciliation Commission. What was that, and how was it used to heal?

Bruce: The Truth and Reconciliation Commission was a commission started by the South African government, headed by Archbishop Desmond Tutu. He won a Nobel Peace Prize and has written a book on this. And it was like a traveling roadshow that went through South Africa after apartheid after Nelson Mandela came to power, and we had our first elections. We were living in a democratic South Africa for the first time.

A lot of bad shit happened during apartheid for want of a better way of putting it, and Mandela was smart enough to know that if we didn't forgive each other, nothing would change.

We might have democracy on paper, but there would still be a lot of hatred and resentment between whites and blacks in South Africa.

So what they did is, and my statistics may not be accurate because it's been a long time since I read precisely the number, but I think they gave everybody a six-month amnesty period. And in that six months, if you'd committed a crime that was for political gain, no matter what it was, whether it was murder or theft, extortion, if it was for the benefit of the country as far as you were concerned, you could come forth, admit your crime and be pardoned. But you would be pardoned on the condition that you made amends for what you had done. So, if you had murdered somebody, you would perhaps have to stand in the Truth and Reconciliation Commission and stand trial and apologize to the parents of the person you murdered or the wife of the person you murdered.

And the idea was that you would get to free your conscience, make amends, and heal the impact you had had in the community by your actions.

And it was controversial; it was like watching the best soap opera you've ever seen in your life. It was moving; touching, and I believe it played a massive role in healing South Africa after our elections in 1994. It was a pretty smart thing to do and ballsy.

Duncan: That idea, we can all hold these commissions in our lives.

Bruce: Exactly. That's what we want to be doing in our own lives, having Truth and Reconciliation Commissions, going to the people we've hurt, the people we've wronged, the people we've lost connection with that we want to have connection with, and healing.

And when you can do that, you have extraordinary relationships.

WHEN THE VIOLIN

When
The violin
Can forgive the past

It starts singing.

When the violin can stop worrying
About the future

You will become
Such a drunk, laughing nuisance

That God
Will then lean down
And start combing you into
His
Hair.

When the violin can forgive
Every wound caused by
Others

The heart starts
Singing.

Hafiz, 14th century Sufi poet and spiritual teacher
Translated by Daniel Ladinsky

I WANT TO FEEL

She has blonde hair. She walks through the door and sits at the head of the table. She's wearing an all-in-one, purple velvet tracksuit. Written on her bottom in capital letters is the word, 'JUICY.'

I'm 21, living in Vancouver, and all I want is to be with her. I spend an entire year trying to impress her. A few days before moving back to England, she agrees to go on a date with me.

"Let's play a game," she says. "It's backgammon but with shots of vodka. Every time you lose a piece, you have to take a shot."

We start to play.

I lean in to kiss her. She kisses back.

We play some more backgammon. We kiss some more.

My mind is not really on the game. She takes one of my pieces; I do a shot of vodka. She takes another, then another, then another, until all of my pieces are gone. I have taken two of hers; she has taken fifteen of mine.

We continue kissing.

We go upstairs to my bedroom, and we start taking each other's clothes off. We're on the bed; I'm so excited. I can't believe this is going to happen.

We begin to have sex, but something isn't right.

No, no, no, no, I think. *Not now, please, not now.*

Stay up! Please, please stay up!

But it gets smaller and smaller and smaller.

I'm trying to do something, *anything.* But everything I try makes it worse.

I look at her and apologize; she seems disappointed. I don't say anything else. We lie there until she falls asleep. Eventually, I do too.

I wake up in the middle of the night. I like her so much. I can't believe she's in my bed lying next to me. She is so beautiful it's ridiculous.

I start to feel some movement down there.

I wake her up.

We start to kiss again.

More movement down there.

We kiss some more.

It's back on!

Thank God for that!

We begin to have sex.

But then it gets smaller again.

"I think I'm going to go home now," she says.

We both get dressed in silence. I walk her across campus back to her apartment. I say goodbye.

I'm wide awake. I don't need sleep; I need answers.

So I walk to the nearest hospital and wait in the reception until a doctor arrives to begin the morning shift. I walk into his office. I close the door behind me. I undo my belt and pull my trousers and underwear down to my ankles.

"What seems to be the problem?" he asks.

I look down, take a deep breath, and say, "I think I've got cancer."

————

I don't have cancer.

But I do leave the surgery with something; a small box of blue pills and the fear that this will happen again every time I like someone.

I'm twenty-one, Viagra is the last thing I need. I know that. But from then onwards, whenever I'm with a girl, I have two choices.

1) Don't take the pill (but be so anxious that it will happen again).
2) Take the pill (but feel completely numb, like a robot; sex is now a process, not an experience).

The choice is easy. I choose disconnection; I choose indifference. I choose results, not rewards, and I have years of meaningless sex with people who are probably wonderful, but I have no idea because I feel nothing.

————

I'm tired of hiding.

I'd prefer to fail at something real than succeed at something fake. So I stop taking them.

But I still have one pill left in my wallet. I can't throw it away. It's my safety net; I have to keep it, just in case.

I go to a music festival called Dekmantel. I'm in the queue about to go through security when I remember that I have a bit of ecstasy in my pocket. I try to move it. The guard sees me, and he asks me to follow him to a curtained-off area. He finds the ecstasy, and he also finds my last blue pill.

"They're both Viagra," I say. "I need them medically."

I feel like I'm close to persuading him, but then he catches himself: "I'm sorry, but you are not convincing me that a green pill, in a plastic bag, in the shape of the Hulk, is medication. You have two choices: one, keep the blue pill and leave the festival or two, throw it in the bin, and you can stay."

No more hiding.

No more safety nets.

No more indifference. I want to feel.

JUDSON BREWER, MD, PHD

Addiction psychiatrist, 20 years
at Yale, MIT, and Brown University
researching how our brains form negative
behavior patterns, bestselling author
of *Unwinding Anxiety*.

*How do we cause ourselves unnecessary suffering? Why
are some people able to move on after challenging
events when others are not? I asked Judson about
a simple but powerful idea.*

Suffering = Pain x Resistance

Duncan: You were taught a formula by a meditation teacher:

Suffering = Pain x Resistance

Judson: Yes. Shinzen Young coined that one. I think it's brilliantly simple. It's not that suddenly, with meditation or awareness, we can make unpleasant things disappear. It's quite the opposite.

We add our own suffering to pain.

So that's where the equation comes in. Pain is there, we can have painful events happen, but when we resist painful things, this is pain x resistance. Now we suffer.

If we stop resisting, if we stop getting caught up in stuff, resistance goes to zero, and therefore suffering goes to zero.

Suffering = Pain x Resistance.

———————

Note: *This is an interesting way to think about suffering. Another way I've heard it described is:*

Pain + Negative Story = Suffering

For example:

Version 1: Your girlfriend dumps you = you feel pain

Version 2: Your girlfriend dumps you + you tell yourself that you're unlovable and you're going to die alone = now you suffer

What If We Just Let It Happen?

Judson: If we're driving a car and we drive the car with one foot on the brake and one foot on the gas, we're not going to get very good gas mileage. And we're going to wear out our brakes pretty quickly.

And wearing out our brakes, think of that as chronic stress, where we're constantly stressed out.

Now what if you take your foot off the brake?

You're not adding any more fuel, but you're more efficient, and your brakes will last a lot longer.

Rather than, "I'm going to *do* this, I'm going to *do* this."

What if we just let it happen?

Not only are we more efficient, but if you take that to its extreme, we move into 'flow', the territory that Dr. Mihaly Csikszentmihalyi talked about in terms of effortless, selfless, timeless, joyful, that type of thing. That sounds pretty good, hey?

ELLIOTT HULSE

Entrepreneur, YouTuber with hundreds of millions
of views, and personal development leader on
a mission to empower others.

*'Work harder,' 'hustle,' 'sleeping's cheating,' 'never quit.'
If you look online or in popular culture, you'll see the
celebration of this mentality. Something I find interesting
is speaking with people whose worldview has changed.
They used to think and act in one way but later abandoned
that approach after seeing its shortcomings.*

An Unresourceful Place

Elliott: Trying to *make* it happen.

That's been a habit of mine. That's how I've gotten to where
I am – by forcing! By grinding! And I'm realizing more and
more how fruitless that is, how many times I've wasted my
energy and then had to do things over again because it wasn't
right because I'm fearfully *going after it* rather than *being* the
thing and allowing it to unfold.

I was proceeding from a place of fear and anger for a lot of my
early life.

"I've got to *prove myself*! I'm going to *do it! No one's* going to
stop me!"

I was able to achieve a lot, but I wasted a lot of energy trying to do things fast – trying to conquer. We use these terms because they're very pleasing to the ego, and they're very pleasing to society: *"Grind!"* and *"Crush It!"* and *"Go hard!"*

And I get it because there's a time you need to do that, but when it's coming from a place of lack, when it's coming from a place of fear when it's coming from a place of anger and having to prove yourself, man, I wasted *a lot* of energy in that place.

It was a very unresourceful place to proceed from.

WALLACE J. NICHOLS, PHD

Marine biologist, bestselling author of Blue Mind: How Water Makes You Happier, More Connected and Better at What You Do.

In 2017, one of my best friends, Nick, was in California. He called me up one day to tell me that he'd gone to a fascinating talk. It was about the neuroscience of how being in or around water affects our mental health. Apparently, the speaker was fantastic, and I needed to interview him. Before he hung up, he said, "Oh, and I bought you a blue marble."

"Thank you so much," I replied. "Why?"

He told me it was a symbol of gratitude, and it represented our blue planet. I followed up on his suggestion, and it was a good one – Wallace J. Nichols was indeed fantastic. But Nick, that was almost five years ago. Where's my marble?

Red Mind, Blue Mind, Grey Mind

Wallace J.: Each of us should become, like you said, familiar with the users' guide to our own brain.

If you ever shopped at IKEA for some furniture and got it home, and it's all in pieces, imagine trying to figure it out without the guide, without that cartoon instruction sheet. You'd be in trouble probably; there'd be parts and pieces and holes and boards and stuff. Well, that's kind of how we've been operating with the human brain. In school, nobody says, "Hey, this is how your brain works, this is how you can hack it, so it works better; here are some tips."

Duncan: That's what I love about having conversations like this; it's like having a toolbox for happiness. After this conversation, a new tool to add to the box is understanding the transformative power of water and being in nature. What are some of the big things that the research has shown? For example, when you're near water, cortisol levels go down, so that's a stress hormone. What other things?

Wallace J.: I think the best way to understand Blue Mind and the role of water is to start with what I call Red Mind, and Red Mind is the opposite of Blue Mind. It's necessary; we do need to get excited, we do need to get angry, we do need to get fired up, to get things done, to survive, to run away. The fight or flight response is natural; it's essential for survival.

But in our modern society, that fight or flight button is being pressed way more than it needs to.

So you open your email, you open a text message, you turn on the TV, you look online, and there's something that's meant to shock you.

That's sort of how our media works, and it's coming from all over the world, so we're overstimulated; the level of psychological stress that we each carry is higher. There's just a lot of input. There's a lot of sensory input; there's a lot more information coming into your brain than your parents had to deal with and their parents and their parents.

You're consuming more information in a day than humans hundreds of years ago consumed, maybe in a month or a year.

Think about that. And you're processing all of that, and you're making sense of it, and you're figuring out what's useful and what's not, you're filtering it. That's our normal base state, and it's not all good, it's not all good for us, it does break us down, it does stress us out, it does tire us out, and we aren't at our best creatively, we are not at our best in terms of relationships.

It puts a strain on things that we agree are important to us.

So that's Red Mind. It's normal; it's chronic, it starts when you wake up in the morning and goes till you put your phone next to your head at night, and then it starts all over again when you wake up and look at your phone, and it's on, screens everywhere.

Blue Mind is when you step away from that – and water helps us make that break more quickly.

You can do mindfulness meditation; you can exercise, but it works better and faster if you add water to it.

If you go for a jog, that's good. If you go for a jog by the river, it will probably get you further into Blue Mind, more quickly into that relaxed state.

If you want to sit in the middle of your room and meditate, that would be nice, but if you sit by the water, you might get to where you want to get a little more quickly.

When we step up to the water, it frees up bandwidth so that visually, the information coming in – that's being processed by the visual centers of our brain – is minimized, simplified.

Looking out at the water, it's interesting, but it's simple.

Now you're not processing words; you're not processing stuff coming off screens.

Auditorily, it's also simplified. The sound of water, a creek, a river, or the waves lapping on the beach is interesting, but it doesn't need much attention. It does not require us to focus. There's no language in that noise; there's no jarring in that noise, no shock, it's calming.

And then somatically, so our bodies, if you're in the water – and you want to be in the water, and you're comfortable – then gravity goes away. You're floating, and the parts of your brain that need to coordinate those two hundred muscles you're using right now to sit upright in that chair get a break.

So all those parts of your brain are getting some bandwidth back.

And what happens is your brain doesn't just go to sleep, it doesn't turn off, it doesn't take a little nap. It does other things that it hasn't been able to do because you've been so focused; you've been all up in the front of your brain, your prefrontal cortex. So the analysis and the processing, the worrying, the second-guessing, that's where we live most of the time.

When you get out to the water, more of your brain is activated in a more distributed fashion; it switches to a different mode, where it's good at other things.

It's not good at focusing on math problems, but it is good at creativity, so when you're in that mode, you have those "Aha!" moments, insights, and connections. People say, "I just wrote a poem, and it just kind of dropped into my mind, almost complete." That's the stuff that happens. When you're urgently trying to weave through traffic, your brain's not writing a poem.

It's not all about poetry, it's about creativity and innovation and connection, but that's the walk-through from Red Mind to Blue Mind.

The third mind that I describe in my book, Gray Mind, is the numbed out, indifferent, mildly depressed, I don't care...

Duncan: Apathy.

Wallace J.: Apathetic, yeah. Pretty useless. Red Mind is useful. Blue Mind is useful. Gray Mind is not so helpful; it's more of a dysfunction.

Blue Mind can help you pull out of that as well.

Water Rehabilitation

Duncan: I watched the short documentary, *Resurface*, which you feature. It's focused on the rehabilitation of army veterans, from amputees to PTSD, and the healing qualities of being out in the surf and the water. I appreciate that you don't want to make big health claims, magic pills, etc. However, just from a visual perspective, somebody would walk into the water in one emotional state, and they'd leave the water differently. Even if it was just temporary, there was a transformation.

So even without the big claims of "It does X, Y, and Z," just seeing someone walk into the water and come out in a different place, someone who was suffering from severe PTSD, it was great to see.

Wallace J.: Yeah, I could tell, you could tell, that film tells many stories, many anecdotes of precisely that, and what's starting to happen is those anecdotes are being collated into long-term studies, and those results are being published. It's really cool to see.

That's One Life Improved

Wallace J.: If one person listens and says, "Wow, I used to love being in the water when I was a kid. I'm stressed out. If I get back in the water, I bet my stress will go down, and I'll be a nicer person, I'll be a happier person, my relationships will be better." If that's what they walk away with from listening to this conversation, wow, that's one life that it's improved.

You don't have to go too far to find proof that this idea is real. And I love it when the studies come together and provide robust evidence that changes our systems, that changes the way we teach, maybe changes the way doctors and nurses do their job.

If water can help people be more creative, reduce stress, manage pain, and help people through the end of their lives, that's just one more set of reasons that we should make sure the water is not polluted.

What My Father Taught Us

Wallace J.: This is what my father taught us, and he didn't teach it through words; he taught us through his actions, and he passed away last year.

A good life, fulfilled life, is one where you're born, you give everything you have, and then you die.

That's it.

That's what he taught us. So I'm in the middle of giving as much as I possibly can, in every way I can. Intellectually, emotionally, spiritually, physically, raising my daughters, my relationship with my wife, my massive family of adopted, biological, and foster brothers and sisters, the environment that I care so much about, animals, the ocean.

The more I give, the better I feel.

And so my dad was right.

DOUGLAS RUSHKOFF

Professor of Media Theory and Digital Economics,
named one of the "world's ten most influential
intellectuals" by MIT, bestselling author
of *Present Shock*.

*It's cool when you're speaking with someone, and they
say something that you're not expecting them to say.
Douglas is a pioneering commentator on media and
technology. We were talking about tech and the digital
world that we live in. Then he said something so simple,
but it was a timely reminder.*

Are We Part of Nature?

Douglas: There's a lot of research that furniture makers in Europe cut down trees depending on which week of the lunar cycle it is because the pores of the wood are open during certain weeks of the lunar cycle and much more closed during another one. So if you cut down when they're open, then more of the sap comes out, or they dry faster, something like that.

People have known these things for thousands of years; it's just whether we accept that human beings are part of nature.

The key to progress may not be trying to continually ignore and override these natural rhythms and cycles of nature but learning how to play with them.

"Happiness is the joy you feel moving towards your potential."

SHAWN ACHOR

"For a long time, it had seemed to me that life was about to begin – real life. But there was always some obstacle in the way. Something to be got through first, some unfinished business, time still to be served, a debt to be paid. Then life would begin. At last, it dawned on me that these obstacles were my life."

ALFRED D'SOUZA

INFINITE GAMES

SIMON SINEK

"I've become very, very interested in the idea of playing in games that have no finish lines. Some games have finish lines – baseball, football. Getting a part is a finish line. You audition, there's a beginning, middle, and end, there's rehearsal and practice, there's showing up for the audition, and you either win or you lose, and then it's over. It's over. That is finite.

"But one's career is infinite. There's no end. Our lives are finite. But 'life' is infinite. People come, and people go, but 'life' continues. Theatre actors come, and actors go, but 'theatre' continues. It's infinite. You don't 'win theatre.' You win a part, but what happens once you get the part?

"The finite game is over; now you enter the infinite game, you have to be able to convert. And the reason this is important, and I've seen this unfortunately so many times…from a young age, all you wanted to do was, "Get to Broadway," and then you get to Broadway, and then what? You've devoted your entire life to one finite goal; when you get there, the immediate response is depression because I've spent fifteen years of my life for this one thing, and I got it, and now I don't know what to do next. Get to Broadway again? It doesn't have the same ambition, it doesn't have the same passion…and this is because these are finite goals.

"There's a lot of studies that have been done with athletes who have finite goals, so "become the greatest X in the world." Andre Agassi was one of these athletes. He wanted to become the greatest tennis player that ever lived. Everyone in his life, he would view them through "How do you help me get to that?" Everything was, "How does this help me get to that?" Everything was a transaction. "How do you help me move to there?"

"And then you know what happens? He achieves it. He became the greatest tennis player in the world, and you know what happened immediately after? Depression.

"Michael Phelps set out to be the most medalled Olympian in history. Do you know what? He achieved it! Do you know what happened immediately after? Depression.

"They spend their whole life working for one goal. Though most will never get it, the few who do, don't know what to do next because their goals were finite. Their goals were finite. And so, there are finite components to your career, but your career should be infinite. Yes, of course, you have to win the finite game, you have to get the part, but immediately when you get the part, now you convert to infinite."[13]

> **Note:** *Personal growth is an example of an 'infinite goal.'*
>
> *Pursuing mastery is an infinite game.*
>
> *You don't ever win mastery.*
>
> *There is no endpoint.*
>
> *You are interested in growth, the pursuit of excellence, the love of the process, rather than a fixation on a desired result or outcome.*

LISA FELDMAN BARRETT, PHD

Professor of Psychology, one of the most-cited scientists in the world, bestselling author of *How Emotions Are Made: The Secret Life of the Brain.*

A friend of mine told me to check out the podcast Invisibilia. She suggested I start with an episode called 'Emotions.' I'm glad I did because that is how I learned about Lisa Feldman Barrett. According to Lisa, our understanding of how emotions work is wrong. Lisa won the Pioneer Award for her revolutionary research on emotion in the brain. These multi-million-dollar awards go to scientists of exceptional creativity.

No Concept for Table, No See Table

Duncan: The thing that made my brain feel weird when I heard you describe it, and correct me if I get any of it wrong, was the parallel between emotions and vision.

With vision, if we didn't have a concept for an object, say, a table or chair, we wouldn't even be able to see that object?

We'd only see bright and dark.

So, for example, I've got this concept, construct, story, whatever you call it, of table-ness. *A table is a flat surface with four legs.* Because I have that concept in my head, I can see tables.

If I didn't have the concept of table-ness in my head, then I wouldn't be able to see the object?

It would just be bright and dark. That's what blew my mind.

Lisa: That's right, if you don't have a concept, if your brain can't make a concept for something, you can't see it.

That may sound unbelievable to people, but your brain is constantly facing a category construction problem. When it receives input from the world or the body, it's not asking, *what is this? It's asking, what is this like? What is this similar to from my past experience?*

And if you don't have past experiences that you can somehow combine to make sense of this sensory input, your brain treats it as noise.

That's why when you hear the sounds of a language that you don't have concepts for, it sounds like noise to you.

That's why when you hear music from a different culture that has a different scale to it, it sounds like noise to you.

My daughter, at some point, was fascinated with dubstep, and I was like, "What is this? This just sounds like noise to me," and then, of course, I was like, "Argh, only old people say that about their kids' music!"

Duncan: If someone's born blind or has a problem with a cataract and later in life, maybe thirty years later, they have the cataract removed, what might happen to that person?

Lisa: Yeah, there are a number of cases where people are either born with cataracts that are sufficiently severe that no input from the eye, from the retina, makes it to the brain and so they're functionally blind, then their cataracts are removed later in life as adults. Or you also have cases where people have corneal damage, which causes the same problem that no light makes it in from the world to the brain. Then at some point, people have, as adults, a corneal transplant.

You would imagine that they'd be able to see immediately upon light entering the retina.

But actually, that's not true; they don't see.

They have to learn to see because they have no prior experience with seeing.

> **Note:** *This is also the case with our emotions. Most of us believe that emotions like fear, sadness, excitement are universal, built into us from birth. It turns out this is not the case.*
>
> *For every emotion category that we have that we think is biologically basic and universal, at least one culture in the world doesn't possess a concept for that emotion. So they don't feel that emotion.*
>
> *If we didn't have a concept for surprise, then we wouldn't be able to feel surprised.*
>
> *If we didn't have a concept for excitement, then we wouldn't be able to feel excitement.*
>
> *If we didn't have a concept for joy, then we wouldn't be able to feel joy.*

KAYPACHA LESCHER

Spiritual practitioner with more than forty years'
experience; uses kundalini yoga, meditation,
and nature for self-renewal.

*It's not easy to be happy if you're pissed off the whole
time. Sometimes we get triggered, and it's not always
clear why. I wanted to find out more.*

Whatever Pisses You Off Is an Aspect of Yourself

Duncan: Whatever pisses you off is a lesson; it's an unexpressed
aspect of yourself. Could you elaborate on that idea?

Kaypacha: Take a simple example like, I want a lot of attention.
When people pat me on the back, smile at me, and tell me I'm
great, it gives me goosebumps all over. *But* my mum and dad or
teachers or preachers told me that that's being egotistical, self-cen-
tered, or narcissistic. I should not demand, expect, or want so
much attention. So then I take that natural desire, and I become
ashamed of it – "I shouldn't be that" or "I shouldn't demand too
much attention" or "I shouldn't yell or scream or shout or dance."

So I stuff that down because I feel bad about it or guilty whenever I express myself.

I see others screaming, shouting, getting attention and people
clapping for them. They become famous or become well-known.

Or maybe it's my brother or sister that gets all the attention, or maybe my spouse or boyfriend or girlfriend or something. They're all charismatic, and everybody adores them and loves them. Then what comes up is, I start to go, "Fuck these guys."

"Look at this person. Look at that person!"

"Who do they think they are?"

"They're so egotistical."

"They think they're so great."

And I start projecting all kinds of negative stuff onto these people who are being allowed to, or succeeding at, living the life that I secretly, or even unconsciously, want for myself.

And so this can be the same with money: "I want lots of money."

"I want power."

Or teachers. We all want to be wise, so we run into a guru or a teacher, and ultimately, we start saying, "You know what, you're full of it."

This is what I call *shadow and projection*.

That what we deny or suppress in ourselves, we make it negative.

And when we see it in somebody else, it triggers us, and we get angry at that person or judge that person.

And so the old saying is, "You spot it. You got it!"

So, if you think somebody's arrogant, guess what? You have some seeds of arrogance yourself, my friend. If you think that somebody is seductive or manipulative, you may be seductive or manipulative yourself.

But this doesn't necessarily mean that it's negative. But when we suppress it, it gets distorted and perverted and becomes negative.

Seductive, let's look at that. We are sexual beings, and this can be a beautiful part of ourselves. But when we judge it and suppress it, then it's like, they're not just naturally a sensual, exotic, erotic person, no, no, no. They're a *slut*, or a *whore*.

We put this negative spin on aspects of human nature that are not necessarily negative.

> **Note**: I know I've personally been guilty of doing this.
>
> A trigger for me was individuals who take advantage of others' good nature – people who focus on 'taking' and 'getting' rather than contributing.
>
> However, this said far more about me than it did about the subjects of my frustration. When I allowed this to upset me the most, I was:
>
> – Still living with my parents
>
> – Eating from the family fridge for all meals
>
> – Only socializing if it was within walking distance of where I lived because I couldn't afford public transport
>
> – Turning up to group dinners an hour late to avoid the meal part and the dreaded "Let's just split the bill," even if you only had a starter and a glass of tap water
>
> – Feeling completely dependent
>
> – Exhausted by it
>
> – Feeling like a charity case
>
> Even though I was proud and insisted on paying my way, I was subtly receiving from all directions: a beer from a friend here, a sofa to crash on there, a meal here, a taxi there.
>
> The reason seeing 'takers' triggered me so much is because I felt like one.

My friends and family cared about me and were probably happy to be able to help. And there are, of course, so many ways to be a giver and to contribute even if you don't have a penny. But in those moments, when I wasn't feeling as confident, and I'd get triggered by seeing selfishness, it was because I felt selfish.

But realizing this was the source of my frustration allowed me to be more forgiving of the people around me and myself.

ISAIAH HANKEL, PHD

Behavioral psychologist, bestselling author of *The Science of Intelligent Achievement: How Smart People Focus, Create and Grow Their Way to Success.*

Do you feel like you're the master of your destiny? I emphasize the word 'feel.' There are so many variables entirely out of our control. But do you feel like you are at least in the driver's seat, behind the wheel of your own life? Put another way, are you the director? When a director films a movie, there are many factors out of their control. Extreme weather. Acts of God. Political unrest. The health of their actors. They must roll with the punches and the challenges as they present themselves. But they can still commit to the process and engage in the creation of the movie. The opposite would be to go through life, never marching to the beat of your own drum. I wanted to speak to Isaiah about how having (or not having) a sense of agency relates to our well-being.

Creative Ownership

Duncan: What do you mean by creative ownership – what does that phrase mean?

Isaiah: Creative ownership; I think this is something that's not talked about enough. What makes people miserable in life is being dependent on other people for their happiness and success.

I don't care who you are, but if you become too dependent on somebody, you'll be miserable.

Some of us are dependent on a boss; we're dependent on one person, maybe a middle manager, whoever it is, one person who controls our career fate. Whether or not we get a promotion, whether or not we go to the office and have a good day, that one person decides our success and happiness – that's dependency, that's not good.

Sometimes people get into relationships and look to that one person for all of their happiness. Whether they had a successful day is if they made that person happy, and they tie everything to that one person. They become utterly dependent on that one person. If that person's mood is down, their mood is down, and this goes on and on in life, personal life, professional life, everything.

So creative ownership is about creating areas of your life, things that you own. It could be a personal project, something like starting a book, starting a podcast, starting a new business, something you own entirely. So that no matter what you're doing, you can experience a sense of growth. You're completely in control over your growth in this area. Nobody else is; you're not dependent on anybody else.

It's very freeing. It opens up a lot of possibilities. It gives you more of an abundant mentality; it opens you up to be more creative.

Duncan: If you have creative ownership, then when you turn up to your relationship or your job, it's a much more empowering position. Rather than being needy, "I need you to fix me."

Isaiah: Yes. And we've all seen that. For example, you see people's parents get a divorce. Before the divorce, they're thirty or forty pounds overweight; not happy, they're miserable. They're not doing any hobbies; they just come home and sit in front of the TV. Then they get divorced, start taking on all these new hobbies, rock climbing, skiing, going out, meeting new people. They lose weight; they get back in shape.

What happened? There's no reason they couldn't have done that before, and the relationship would have been a lot better. But they become codependent and rely on each other for their happiness. One person couldn't do what they wanted to do because of wanting to keep the other person happy. The other person couldn't do what they wanted because they were worried about upsetting the other person.

So they weren't who they needed to be; they weren't independent, and being independent makes you the best possible person in relationships. It makes you the best possible worker in businesses. Companies know this too. That's why many companies allow you to have a certain percentage of your time where you can work on whatever you want to work on; they're making you less beholden to doing the same old routine nine-to-five work. Independence is freeing. It makes people creative; it makes them work harder. It makes them better people overall.

Experiencing Growth in at Least One Area of Your Life

Duncan: You posted a video on YouTube explaining that your previous thoughts and teachings about happiness were wrong. Tell me about that; what was that video, and what was the update?

Isaiah: One of the prime human needs that we all have is growth.

In my first book, I said that happiness is experiencing growth in every area of your life, and I think that was wrong.

Happiness is experiencing growth in *any area* of your life, not every area.

The mistake that many of us make is that we make our lives one-dimensional. We're just focused on business, or just focused on family, or just focused on whatever hobby. If we have a bad day in that area, if we don't experience growth in that one area, there goes our happiness.

So really, what you need to do is not tie your identity only to one thing; you need to have multiple things happening in your life.

Maybe you go to the gym and take care of your health; maybe you have friends and family or working on a business or a side project. Have multiple areas where you can experience growth daily, so no matter what happens, you're experiencing growth in at least one area of your life. And that's happiness.

It doesn't have to be in every area. It's *any* area.

Emotions Travel Through Networks Like Flu

Duncan: Each positive person you surround yourself with increases your chances of being positive by eleven percent. Not bad, eleven percent.

However, each negative person you let into your life more than doubles your chances of being negative. That's quite a big difference.

Isaiah: It is, yeah. People study how emotions travel through networks, and epidemiologists can see that emotions fluctuate through groups of people and travel the same way that influencer does.

So when you see negative information, you're around a negative person, you're going to become negative because your brain loves it; it's super sticky to your brain.

"Consumers of negative news, not surprisingly, become glum: a recent literature review cited 'misperception of risk, anxiety, lower mood levels, learned helplessness, contempt and hostility towards others, desensitization.' And they become fatalistic."

STEVEN PINKER, PHD

YOU'RE WEIRD.
CONGRATULATIONS!

I'm not a wizard, but if I did go to the same school as Harry Potter, I know what boarding house I'd be put in: it would be the house for the brave, the heroes.

I'm sure most of you know this, but there are four options: one house for the brave, one for the baddies – they're all a bit evil in that one, one house for the intelligent people, and then last of all, there's Hufflepuff.

This is the house for all the…others. I'm not entirely sure what their thing is, but they're all pretty weird.

I want to confirm what I already know to be the case, so I go onto the Harry Potter website. I click a button and begin to answer a personality test. After the last question, the page turns yellow:

"Congratulations, you're a Hufflepuff."

Absolutely not.

I close the internet browser. I wait ten seconds; then I open it up again. I return to the website, and I start a brand-new test, but this time around, I lie. Every time I want to answer one way, I select the opposite answer. After the last question, the page turns yellow:

"Congratulations, you're a Hufflepuff."

This is bullshit. It has no idea the type of person I am.

What would you do if you wanted to prove how brave you were?

Me? I decide I'm going to join the army so I can fight in a war!

I'm already online, so I look up their website and apply. The next day, I received an email. It's a short message; it just has an address in the north of the city, and it says to come next Thursday at 6 pm.

The day arrives, I'm curious, nervous, and excited, but most of all, I'm determined. By the time I leave, there will be no doubt in anyone's mind how brave I am.

I get to the address. There's a building. Above the doorway is a sign saying 'Registration' and a queue of people. I join the line. In front of me is a man. He's covered in green and brown paint; he has moss, bark, and leaves stuck to his clothes.

I put out my hand. "Hi, I'm Duncan."

"*Hissssssssss*," he says. "I'm a tree…a treeeeeeeeeee."

He turns back around.

I get to the front of the queue. A lady asks me to pay $2, then she hands me a rubber sword and informs me that I now have insurance.

I exit through a door at the back of the building, leading directly onto a park. There are between one hundred and eighty to two hundred orcs, goblins, knights, kings, queens, wizards, and demons standing on the grass.

A man in full armor approaches. He has a plumed helmet, like something out of the film *Gladiator*, and a second man walks directly behind him, holding his cape.

The main guy is sniffing the air. "Cheese...cheese...I smell cheese?" he says.

"Don't you mean blood, sire?" the second man responds.

"Soon...yes. *Very* soon." Then he walks away, still sniffing the air.

A man with seven human skulls hanging from his belt explains the rules to us and informs us that the sound of a horn will indicate the start of the battle.

"When you hear the horn for a second time," he says, "the battle is over, and you must lower your weapons." He assigns us to a team – one hundred people on one side of the park, facing one hundred people on the other.

The horn sounds, and we begin to charge.

I have no game plan, no strategy. I'm running as hard as I can. Adrenaline is flooding through my body. I begin swinging my arms and making various stabbing and chopping motions. I see one of the enemies; I lift my sword, spin on my heel to create momentum, and decapitate him.

Or at least, I would have if my sword wasn't rubber.

The guy breaks character and begins rubbing his neck. "*Not cool,* dude! Not cool."

"I'm so sorry," I say. "I have no idea why I did that. It's my first time. I'm really sorry."

I rejoin the battle.

A few minutes later, I feel something bounce off me. I look around, but there's nothing there.

"Pssst."

"Psssst."

"*Pssssst.*"

A man dressed in an emerald gown is pointing at something on the ground.

"What is it?" I say.

He grabs something from his leather saddle bag and makes an underarm motion towards me; a ball made from foam bounces off my thigh.

I look at him in confusion.

"It's a spell!" he says. "I hit you with a spell."

"Ohh, okay." I put one of my arms behind my back.

"And *another* one," he says.

"Why?"

"I hit you twice," he says. "Two spells, so you lose two limbs."

I lift my left leg and hop away from him.

I can't fight in this state; I need my limbs back.

I have two options. Option one: I lie motionless on the ground until a healer arrives by my side.

"Abra Cooobara Cooobara,

Lacka Lacka Lacka,

Hyster-Rista Hyster-Rista,

Salamander Salamander Salamander,

Banda Panda."

I'll get back one of my limbs for every thirty seconds of incantations they recite.

I look around, but there's no medic in sight.

That only leaves me option two: try and make my way over to the other side of the park, where there's a healing bay.

I must bow my head in submission, lift my sword high into the air to show that I am no longer a threat, and walk by touching my left foot to my right foot, then my right foot to my left foot, heel to toe, in an unbroken chain.

Heel to toe, heel to toe, heel to toe, heel to toe.

It's taking a long time.

Heel to toe.

Probably the least efficient way I've ever tried to get somewhere.

Heel to toe.

But it gives me time to breathe and time to think.

I look around the battlefield at the faces of my comrades, my brothers and sisters, my weird, really, really weird brothers and sisters, running around, doing their thing. I realize that, right now, there is nowhere else that I would rather be.

You're weird. Congratulations!

Don't pretend you're not.

And it dawns on me: I want to be, I'm excited to be, I *get to be*...

A Hufflepuff!

MASTIN KIPP

Recognized as a "thought leader for
the next generation" by Oprah Winfrey.
His work has helped over two million people
in more than 100 countries, bestselling
author of *Claim Your Power*.

*It's great to identify the habits and practices that increase
happiness. But I also wanted to better understand what
prevented many people from feeling joy. One thing is
emotional trauma. A man who is leading a public
conversation around trauma is Mastin Kipp.*

If You Step on a Nail, What Would You Do?

Mastin: Lots of things create trauma, and what happens is that,
early in someone's process, they cope with it in what I'll call
low-level coping. So it might be drugs, alcohol, promiscuity – the
opioid crisis is massive in America. There are many different
ways to cope with it that are not good for the body.

But then, without addressing it, you upgrade your life. And you
have *high-level coping* like a yoga class, biohacking, different
ways of putting butter in your coffee, or measuring your sleeping performance, whatever it is. And getting those data points
is important, but no biohack will out-hack emotional trauma,
which is emotional wounding.

I'm a big fan of all the things that we've talked about: meditation and green juicing, and yoga, but without doing the trauma work, it becomes high-level coping.

If you step on a nail, what would you do?

You would feel it, it would be painful, and then you would look at it and assess how bad it is. If it's bad enough, you go to the emergency room. If it's not that bad, you get the first aid kit, and you would clean it out. And if you went to the emergency room, they would clean it out. They would put some stitches on it, maybe give you some pain medicine, say stay off it for a week or two, standard RICE protocol: rest, ice, compression, elevation. Make sure to keep the wound clean, and then over a few weeks or a month or so, you would be back on your feet, do a little bit of rehab, and then go about your life. And ten years later, you wouldn't be sitting there going, "God damn it, that one time with that nail in my foot!" You wouldn't be worried about it; you would just be moving on. Maybe you'd see a scar every once in a while.

But that's not how we do things emotionally. What we do is we hit a nail.

"No, no, no, I'm good."

"I'm not going to look at it."

"Don't talk about it."

"You can't acknowledge a negative; Voldemort will show up!"

And "Only positive things!"

"I am healthy! I am vibrant! I can walk with *ease!*"

Even though there's pain.

And we ignore it, and depending on how long you ignore it, don't be surprised if one day you look down and your whole left leg has gangrene because you've ignored a wound.

And the problem with emotional trauma is it's, for now, invisible, so it's really hard to see it fester because it grows on you, slowly. These emotions can become very gripping, and you can say that everything's great, but then one, two, or three things change in your life, and BAM! There you are, back in the feeling again. So it's something that you have to maintain vigilance around.

The Goal Is to Understand That Trauma Is Like a Virus

Mastin: If you go to the monkey forest in Bali, if you go anywhere where normal mammals are doing normal mammal things, they're eating each other alive, and they're committing sexual assault all the time! And somehow, human beings have evolved out of that muck and formed things like law and values.

We've evolved out of this very violent world. We've evolved from a lot of violence and trauma of the past.

Epigenetics has now shown that trauma gets passed down generationally. So it would make sense from a biological perspective why there is war and rape and these types of things. Not endorsing it, but if you look at the past of what we've evolved from, that's normal, and so we're flushing out these values that are no longer necessary, like racism. There was a time when racism was probably a good survival response, thousands and thousands of years ago when the tribe was coming to rape and pillage your village. Now, it's just an echo of a past that doesn't serve us anymore. So that's what I mean by yesterday's medicine has become today's poison.

There was a time when these things were so commonplace. And now, with what's happening with technology and all that, we're learning about how the body works. Epigenetics, genomics, all the somatic and trauma work, all this inner stuff we're starting to be able to weigh and measure. We've never had access to things like this before, and we're beginning to see, "Wow, we can actually get along."

And if you think about it from an evolutionary perspective, human beings developed the ability to cooperate and have empathy and compassion. Those are evolutionary benefits because we need to be together and co-regulate for our survival. We can't do it on our own.

And so, if you look at it purely from the sense of evolution, we've evolved from a very traumatic history. Things are not awesome right now – I'm not saying things are awesome, but compared to how they were ten or twenty thousand years ago, it's a lot better. Even a hundred years ago, women couldn't vote, black people couldn't vote; many things weren't possible a hundred years ago. So there's been rapid progress if you think about it in the context of thousands and thousands of years; in the last hundred years, we've made rapid progress.

We still have a *long* way to go, but it's still the trauma work, and I feel like part of our evolution to whatever we're becoming next in our planetary societies, one of the things that have to happen to sustain that is we have to learn how to heal this trauma thing so that we're not acting like our predecessors. We have to learn how to collaborate.

And so that's why whenever I do this work, I'm not endorsing anyone's specific behavior and certainly am not endorsing the values of racism and xenophobia. But in the context of biology and evolution, it makes sense. When you can see it through that lens, you can start to have compassion for people who have blind spots around this.

And when someone feels seen, heard, loved, and recognized, they drop a lot of those defensive values. Most people don't believe what they say they believe; they say what they believe to fit into a tribe.

If you give them a better option to fit into another tribe where they're accepted for who they are, then the truth starts to emerge.

So we're in the middle of this massive upheaval and identification of all the wounds we've endured emotionally for a very long time, and that's why the world seems like it's going crazy right now.

All these wounds have always been there, but we're just more aware of it and more connected than ever before because of the internet and technology. More connected to the resources, more connected to the outcomes, more connected to what's possible. But also more connected to the wounding and the hurt.

And so that's what's happening today. You're seeing women speaking up in the #MeToo movement. It's so necessary; it's so needed. You see the Time's Up movement evolve. You're seeing Supreme Court nominees being stopped and paused and victims being listened to. It's a big, big deal. You're seeing influential people in Hollywood and entertainment media having reckonings because the time has come for this trauma conversation to emerge. It's happening in front of our very eyes. It's incredible to see it on such a large scale but to solve the problem, the goal is to understand that trauma is like a virus – everyone has it.

So we can jail certain people and not tolerate certain values, but if we want to get through this process, this is when we need to practice the idea of 'love your neighbor as yourself.' Love your enemy. Martin Luther King said that – he was quoting Jesus – these are timeless ideas. It's more important now than ever.

Witness It, but Don't Linger in It

Mastin: Part of healing shame is witnessing it but not lingering in it. That's the hard part.

Duncan: Okay, so that's key: witness it, talk about it, but rather than going to therapy every week to dig it up again, dig it up again, to recognize it, to put it in the light, and then let it go?

Mastin: Yeah, because what happens is there are phases. When someone's traumatized, and they hold it by themselves and finally share it, there's this relief of, "Oh my god, I'm not alone." They get a lot of praise and connection from that experience.

However, it's kind of like getting sober. Once you get sober, that's a huge milestone. But at some point, you go, "And what else? I'm sober, and now what?"

And that's when the purpose, fulfillment, growth, contribution, and all the gifts of sobriety start to come in. And the same thing is true when you're healing from trauma.

I don't like to use the word *victim* because I think that word has been so overused. So I'm not going to use that word, but what I will say is, when someone experiences trauma, they become a lot more passive in how they engage with the world. They get more on the defense than they do being proactive.

Once your wound has been witnessed and validated, staying in that long-term creates commiseration, which is more healthy than holding it all by yourself. But commiserating only, reliving it only, and blaming people only, keeps you stuck at a certain level.

At some point, you have to take a more proactive approach to how your life will move forward. Once it's witnessed and validated and heard and seen and felt, you say, "And now, I'm in charge of how I respond moving forward, that's on me!" So I want to be more proactive in my response and start to realize that no matter what somebody did to me, I was victimized back then, but that does not prevent me from being proactive in how I respond moving forward.

But you can't just go straight into that. That's what happens; people say, "Oh yeah, just reframe it, and move forward."

No.

The wound has to be witnessed, but it then has to be sown up and healed.

Because otherwise, you're harboring that and harping on it and bonding over the wound only. One of my mentors, Caroline Myss, has a term for that; she calls it *woundology*, where all you do is speak wound.

"It's their fault."

"They did this to me."

"Always this, never that."

And that puts you more at a passive stance or passive passenger seat in your life, versus realizing you're the driver and you can be far more proactive, and it's safe to be proactive. But it's a process to get there.

Design Your Environment

Mastin: It's all about the environment.

The environment you're consistently in will be far more impactful on your long-term results than any mindset you try to maintain.

I'll give you a basic example: there's a place in America called Dunkin' Donuts, and it's a donut shop. If you lived in and never left Dunkin' Donuts, no mindset or willpower will help you lose weight. Maybe you go on a hunger strike, but most people would cave and probably give themselves diabetes if they live inside Dunkin' Donuts. Even if their whole mindset said, "I'm thin, I'm healthy, I'm doing my exercises inside here," it wouldn't happen for most people. So you want to make sure that you're in a positive and healthy environment.

ANNE KREAMER

Former Executive Vice President for Nickelodeon,
author of *Risk/Reward: Why Intelligent
Leaps and Daring Choices Are the Best Career
Moves You Can Make.*

Anne has been at the forefront of the media world since the beginning of her career. In the late 1970s and into the 80s, she distributed and co-produced Sesame Street. A few years later, she helped launch SPY magazine, described as "the most influential magazine of the 1980s." In the 90s, she became the Worldwide Creative Director for Nickelodeon.

Sometimes I Just Do Nothing at All

Anne: In my research, I conducted three big national surveys with J. Walter Thompson, trying to get a hundred-thousand-foot snapshot of what people were feeling about their working lives, and the group of people that I called the *Pioneers* were the most economically, financially successful; they made seventeen percent more money than everybody else. But what was interesting about them was they did several things that were different. One of the things that these pioneers did was they answered, "Sometimes I just do nothing at all," and almost everybody else said they work all the time.

And I profoundly believe that you can't have new creative output in any aspect of your life unless you've had fulfilling input.

And that could be, for me, it would be going out for a walk in the park, or painting or gardening or hanging out, whatever it is, something that nourishes your emotional, spiritual well.

And the most successful people by the measurable benchmark of money, the Holy Grail in America, respected that.

BARRY SCHWARTZ, PHD

Professor of Psychology, TED Talks viewed by
millions, author of *The Paradox of Choice:
Why More Is Less. How the Culture of Abundance
Robs Us of Satisfaction.*

*In his 2004 book and TED Talk 'The Paradox of Choice,'
Barry tackled one of the great questions of modern life.
Why are we witnessing a near-epidemic of depression
amongst societies of great abundance? Nations where
individuals are offered more freedom and choice than
ever before. Conventional wisdom suggests that the
more choice we have, the better. Dr. Schwartz argues
the opposite. He's made a compelling case that the
abundance of options in today's world is making us
miserable. Barry is a goldmine of wisdom and big ideas.
I wanted to use this opportunity to explore a few topics
with him.*

Fixed Mindset vs. Growth Mindset

Barry: My explanation of it, I should make clear is speculative,
but nonetheless. Most of us think that how intelligent you are
is fixed. Some people win the lottery, the genetic lottery, and
some lose it; some people are smart, and some are not, and that's
it. Then the question is, "How close can you come to realizing
your potential?" which is limited by some piece of your biology.

So, you know, that could be true. There's no reason why in principle, that's not true. But a psychologist named Carol Dweck has done some very important work with kids, showing that kids have two different approaches when they go to school.

One kind of kid is interested in demonstrating their ability, and the other is interested in increasing their ability.

Now, this doesn't make much difference in kindergarten, first grade, but in second grade, third grade, you start getting stuff to do that you get wrong, you get math problems that you can't do.

And the kids who want to demonstrate their ability respond to failure – getting things wrong – badly. They avoid challenges, and they do what they can to get approval.

The kids who are interested in getting smarter want to seek challenges. Every mistake they make is an opportunity to learn.

In second grade-ish, around second grade, you have these two groups of kids who look pretty much the same. Then the achievement-oriented kids stay flat, and the mastery-oriented kids go up. And what happens is that they get more and more different over time.

Now, why does this happen? It turns out that achievement-oriented kids have what Dweck calls a 'fixed' naive theory of intelligence. They have the theory of intelligence that I just described to you: "This is how smart we are; we can't get smarter, so why don't I just get as many pats on the head as I can?"

The mastery-oriented kids have what she calls an 'incremental' theory of intelligence (or growth mindset): "Intelligence is not fixed, you can get smarter, and damn it, that's my mission!"

So, here's a case where if you believe that intelligence is fixed, you will not challenge kids, and the result will be that intelligence *is* fixed.

Because you don't get smarter unless you try to get smarter, and if everyone thinks you can't get smarter, no one will try to get smarter. The result will be that nobody does get smarter.

People Who Are Out to Get the Best

Barry: When I give talks about the problem of too much choice, one of the points I make is that the problem is especially significant for people who are out to get the best; I call them *maximizers*. Because if you're out to get the best, you have to look at every possibility, and when there are hundreds of options, it becomes completely daunting. Eventually, you stop, pick something, and you're convinced that something else you hadn't gotten around to looking at would be better.

Duncan: The grass is greener.

Barry: Which means you're not satisfied with what you've got. Well, I have a cartoon from *The New Yorker* magazine that I show to illustrate this, of a young woman wearing a college sweatshirt and the sweatshirt says:

BROWN

But My First Choice Was Yale

I don't know how many people watching this will know what this even refers to. But these are two extremely elite American universities. And you look at it, and you laugh, but the thing to appreciate is how sad it is; to imagine that what's on the sweatshirt is also in this woman's head. She's at Brown, a spectacular institution, and she spends four years at Brown thinking she'd be better off at Yale, and you know what? She's not going to get nearly as much out of Brown as Brown has to offer because every day, she's going to get out of bed saying,

"Oh, I wish I was at Yale, oh, I wish I was at Yale." The result, again, is self-fulfilling.

"How was Brown?"

"It was okay."

If she had gone with a different sweatshirt that said, "Wow! I'm in Brown!" it would have been spectacular. Not just because she thinks it's spectacular. If she has that enthusiasm, she's going to suck it dry of everything that it has to offer instead of passively crawling through the four years to get to the other side and get a job as an investment banker or some damn thing.

So it's very, very powerful. The construal effect (how we perceive and interpret something) is extremely powerful, and in general, we underestimate its importance.

Is It Inevitable for Us to Dislike Our Work?

Duncan: In your latest book, you reference quite a staggering statistic. A quarter of a million people were surveyed across one hundred and forty countries, and the results are pretty alarming.

Barry: They are. To summarize, roughly ten percent of people are really engaged by their work.

Ninety percent are either unengaged – they're just mailing it in, putting in their time, and punching a clock – or they're actively disengaged. In other words, they hate going to work every day.

And the thing that's so striking about this is that this is what we spend at least half our waking lives doing. The question is, "Is it inevitable that we have to spend half our waking lives doing something we don't want to do in a place where we don't want to be?"

There's nothing inevitable about it at all.

And so the question is, can you think about re-visioning work so that it remains productive and profitable and, at the same time, people want to show up every day? They feel like they're going to learn something when they show up. They're going to be challenged. They're going to have some control over what they do. They're going to get some meaning out of their activity.

The evidence is that when you create jobs like this, you increase productivity, not decrease it. So it's better for the boss, and it's better for the employee, which makes you wonder why the hell work isn't organized in this way?

BETTER THAN YESTERDAY

How can I be better today than I was yesterday?

This is one of the most influential questions in my life; it acts as my guide. I'm not that motivated by setting loads of distant goals – I prefer having a reliable system, and my system is: *better than yesterday.*

I want to be better today than I was yesterday.

If I can just focus on compounding that day after day, week after week, month after month, then I have no idea what type of growth is possible; but that is exciting.

Einstein described compound interest as "the most powerful force in the universe." So I'm interested less in goals and more in applying the power of compounding to my personal growth.

Better than yesterday.

I don't have any tattoos, but I've thought about getting one that says BetTY or BETTY. I haven't decided yet if that's inspired or an awful idea.

I can't remember where I heard the following analogy – it may have been Tony Robbins. If you look at nature, nature is in two states: everything is growing or dying.

If you look at a plant, it is either growing or dying.

Humans are part of nature, and the same rule applies to us. We are growing, or we're dying.

If we spend our time sitting around, consuming loads of rubbish content, and talking shit about other people, we are slowly dying. We're just withering away.

So how can you be better today than you were yesterday? It could be by having a great conversation, listening to an audio-book, watching a documentary, doing something for a friend. There are countless possibilities.

When we feel like we're growing, we feel alive.

DAVID MELTZER

Had a net worth of over $120M, then he lost it all.
Then he made it back again.
Award-winning humanitarian and bestselling
author of *Connected to Goodness*.

David grew up poor. All he wanted was to make a load of money to buy his mum a house and a car. He achieved his dream; he bought the house. Then more homes. A golf course. A ski mountain. He had a net worth of over $120M. Then he lost everything; every single penny – they even took his mum's house. But that's not the end of the story; he made it all back again. He became the CEO of the world's most notable sports agency before co-founding one of the world's leading sports and entertainment marketing agencies. Although his business success is interesting, it wasn't why I wanted to speak with him. The thing I found more intriguing was his mindset.

Not Enough, Just Enough, More than Enough

Duncan: Three types of energy states that people often live in. Could you share them?

David: Yeah. One is the world of *not enough*, and that's – it doesn't matter how much you have; it's a mindset of living in a world of "I need more, I need more, I never have enough."

Then there's the world of *just enough*, and a majority of people live in that world. "I just have enough, I just got enough, if I just could do this...."

Duncan: Would that be a perfect example of having enough money until the end of the month, but they're always living paycheck to paycheck?

David: Perfect example and they limit how much they can give to others because of thinking they only have *just enough* for themselves to get by, food, housing. Many Americans live in a world of *just enough*, and I lived there. "If I just had enough to buy my mum a house and a car." That was my world – *just enough*.

And then I started moving to the world of *not enough* even though I made *so* much; there was just not enough, I needed more and more and more, different things and more and more, and it's so empty.

But then, the world of actually *more than enough*, and there are so many examples. There's an island of two hundred thousand people who live and survive off of trash. But they live in a world of *more than enough*. They created a complete universe where everyone has more than enough of everything for everyone.

Kenya, where I do a lot of work in the Bogani in the Masai Mara, it's amazing; everyone's smiling. It's a world of *more than enough* for everyone. They create all types of different systems.

That abundance, that philosophy of enough of everything for everyone, allows you to get into the flow.

MICHAEL PORT

Former actor (*Pelican Brief, Sex and The City, Law & Order*), bestselling author of six books, co-founder & CEO of Heroic Public Speaking.

"I look like a cop and a serial killer." So when the role to play a cop who is secretly a serial killer came along, it looked like Michael's big moment. It was the lead in a movie alongside Morgan Freeman. But unfortunately for Michael, they found someone else who had even more of a serial killer vibe.

Fear of rejection weighs so many of us down; it imprisons us. Few professions have to deal with rejection as regularly as actors do. So I thought, who better to discuss this topic with? Michael is also one of the only former actors to be a New York Times bestselling business author.

The Internal Critics and the External Critics

Michael: Anybody can tear something down. I'm not talking about that; that's the general modus operandi on Facebook, on Twitter – break things down, don't build anything, just break them!

But there are two types of critics.

There are the internal critics and the external critics.

And we fear the external critics significantly when the internal critics are very loud.

And they say, "I'm not enough."

"I don't know enough."

"What do I have to say that hasn't been said before?"

"I'm just not enough."

That's what they say.

And if those voices are loud, then the voices outside, the ones who like to push people down just to lift themselves up, you know those types?

Duncan: Yeah, "BOOO! Get off the stage! You suck!"

Michael: Yeah, it's like they 'boo' the best baseball player in the history of the world because he strikes out once! Like, what? You get these guys who haven't run around the block in twenty years who are going, "You're a bum! You suck. Go home!"

This guy trains twelve hours a day, all day long, and you're telling him he's a bum? Haha, I don't get it!

But that baseball player, performer, CEO, anybody at the top, if they spend their time criticizing themselves, then those voices on the outside will be too loud and too overwhelming.

So our job is to do what we can to silence, or at least turn down the volume on the voices inside our head.

We will question ourselves. I think that's very difficult to eliminate entirely. I did a podcast interview yesterday, and afterward, I was like, "Ahhh, I feel I was kind of, I was not really clear, and I didn't like it." My fiancée said, "Michael, I thought it was one of your best."

I'm like, "Oh, then I suck if *that* was one of my best!"

She's like, "No, Michael, you're an idiot."

I'm like, "I know, I'm an *idiot!*"

Duncan: Haha

Michael: I don't think those feelings go away all the time, but if we can quiet them down, then we don't worry about the external critics as much. Then we are willing to take more risks, go out on a limb, play different roles, share all the things we stand for, not pigeonhole ourselves, and ask for the things we want.

Because if somebody says no, we don't take it so personally.

ENOUGH

MARISA PEER

"I've been a therapist for a long time, but I realized very early on with all my clients and patients that they all had the same problem: they didn't ever think they were enough. Whether they came in with a drug addiction, a shopping addiction, a food addiction, a hoarding addiction, they all went back to the same thing: 'I'm not enough.' Some of my clients were movie stars, Olympic athletes, others maybe school teachers, but 'I'm not enough' is a universal problem that we pick up very early in our lives because we start to compare ourselves to other people… We start to buy into this belief, 'I'm not enough,' and it is the biggest problem I see in the Western world.

"If you think you're not smart enough, attractive enough, interesting enough, intelligent enough, loveable enough; if you have issues with shopping, eating, hoarding, drinking, even binging out on Netflix to hide from the feeling of not being enough… Write 'I am enough' on your mirror in lipstick, eyeliner, or a marker pen, put it on your fridge in fridge magnets, put it all over your house… When you know you're enough, you know what's so amazing? You give the whole world permission to also know that you're enough. And when you think you're not enough? People pick up what you believe about you. You are what you believe. You make your beliefs, and then your beliefs make you. So if you make your belief, 'I'm enough,' I promise you, I guarantee you, it will change your entire life."[14]

IAIN MCGILCHRIST, MD

Neuroscientist, psychiatrist, bestselling author of *The Master and His Emissary: The Divided Brain and the Making of the Western World.*

I wanted to understand better the difference between the right hemisphere and the left hemisphere of our brains and how those differences affect our lives. The world's foremost expert on this subject is Dr. Iain McGilchrist.

Left Brain, Right Brain, Pop Psychology's Big Mistake

Duncan: One central point that you emphasize is that there's absolutely nothing wrong with the left hemisphere – the left hemisphere isn't the baddy. It isn't about getting rid of the left hemisphere – but it doesn't know its limitations.

It's a wonderful tool, it's a great servant, but the danger is that we're living in a society where we've elevated it to the role of the master.

That's the issue: we're putting it in a position that it should not be?

Iain: Exactly! And that's why the book bears the title, *The Master and His Emissary.* The image in the title is that the left hemisphere is a very good servant if it does what it's asked to do.

But the trouble is that it only too quickly thinks it knows more than the right hemisphere, which in reality knows more.

It literally does; that's not a figure of speech. In a literal sense that can be entirely substantiated neurologically, the right hemisphere knows more. It takes in more, attends more, judges better, perceives better, and is more in touch with reality than the left hemisphere.

Interestingly, in pop psychology, the version of things is that the left hemisphere is this rather dull accountant-like figure that is at least reliable. Whereas the right hemisphere tends to be temperamental, a bit pink and fluffy, very creative, but needs anchoring by that good solid left hemisphere. Well, it turns out that's not the case at all.

In every respect, the right hemisphere is more reliable, more down to earth, more "Well, it might be like this, but it might be like that." Ramachandran calls it the devil's advocate; in other words, it's the one that can see "There might be another way of seeing this."

Whereas the left hemisphere, once it's stuck on an idea, it's absolutely stuck on that idea. So we get people who are very much fixed in a worldview in which they think they know everything because they don't know very much. And they can't be dislodged from it. That's a worry.

The Dangers of Left Brain Thinking

Duncan: If I was someone listening to this, why does this matter? Why should I care?

Iain: Well, you come across it every day in the way things are more and more bureaucratized.

Essentially, the left hemisphere way of thinking is bureaucratic mentality.

And so, just trying to do something that has a human element to it is increasingly difficult because it has to follow a flow diagram, and it has to fit in the boxes. Having conversations with people over the telephone when something goes wrong, most people will have this experience. You need to talk to your bank, the telephone company, or somebody else. They've got a script they're working from where the actual individual circumstances you're in don't fit this, and they're not answering your point because there's no enmeshing with these two. That's very simple.

But on a much higher level, what it means is that we think we know how to do things, but in doing what we believe is the logical thing, we make things worse.

So it looks logical to go into the Gulf and stabilize a situation that appears volatile; in fact, what we do is massively destabilize.

We think we can control the stock markets – many Nobel prize-winning economists thought this – so there will never be another crash. As soon as they made these hubristic pronouncements, there was an almighty crash.

We protect children from danger, and we make them vulnerable.

We think that the only way to educate a child is to put lots of information into them; by doing that, we drive out the independence of thinking, which is the point of education in itself.

We protect ourselves from germs because it looks logical, and we make ourselves so vulnerable that we're constantly falling ill.

These are just simple examples in our daily life of how an apparently rational way of thinking – that just sees one little thing and goes for it – leaves out all the complexity of the big picture, which you really ought to take into account if you're going to understand how to behave as a rational person.

The Pursuit of Happiness

Duncan: You said, with all due respect to the American constitution, you can't pursue happiness; the more you pursue it, the more it runs from you. Happiness is a byproduct of forgetting yourself.

Iain: There's such a thing as happiness, of course, and there's such a thing as fulfillment, but they don't come from being themselves pursued. Much as the best way to enjoy sleep is not to have a plan to "Go to sleep now!" You will go to sleep when you're ready to go to sleep, and the more you force yourself to go to sleep, the less you'll do. So it's a little like that.

It comes as a byproduct of forgetting about yourself or about pursuing happiness. It comes from the most surprising places. Often it comes from things that could be frustrating, for example, overcoming obstacles.

One might think that fulfillment and happiness came from there being no obstacles, a life that didn't have its downsides. It could never happen, but it would be impossible to have fulfillment or happiness in that world.

Nothing can be detached from what we think of as its opposite, but it's not its opposite; it's part of it. It's a bit like, think of an iron bar that is a magnet, and you say, "I don't like the south pole. I only like the north pole. I'm going to cut the south pole off!" You don't get rid of the south pole; you just shorten the magnet. Life is like this.

Or, like a circle, if you go far enough around it to get away from where you are, you end up coming back to the same thing. A thing and its opposite are bound up with one another. So, fulfillment is often paradoxical in that way.

No-Input Tuesdays

Duncan: What is a call to action, even if it moves the needle forward just that extra couple of percent?

Iain: Well, I suppose you're asking for something practical that each person can do, and that's easy enough to answer: stop doing quite a lot of things that you think are important, then you'll discover what is important.

So the first thing to do is to create an area of space or an area of time in the day when you absolutely don't do any of the things you think are vital to existence.

So stop constantly talking, communicating.

Create a space for peace, and listen.

And don't expect to hear anything, to begin with; carry on until you do. When you do, it'll be very worthwhile hearing it.

So that's a practical, simple thing that you can incorporate into your life.

Duncan: About five years ago, I realized that I was always in 'doing' mode. I would wake up, check my phone, reply to emails, meeting, meeting, doing, doing, doing, doing, doing.

So I started this thing called No-Input Tuesdays. Every Tuesday morning until about one or two in the afternoon, I have a four-hour window where I'll sit somewhere without any input. No computer, no phone, no music. All I have is a pen and paper.

At first, you might (like I did) twiddle your thumbs, and you might get bored. On the surface, it seems like, "What are you doing? That's so unpractical, it's such a waste of time," but hands down, my biggest "Aha!" moments, breakthroughs, "Do this with the business," "Speak with that person," and moments of pure clarity and total calm have always come in that block...

this massive vacuum of empty space, because we never allow ourselves that space.

It's been one of the biggest game-changers in my life. I love it. I often recommend it to others, especially if they feel constantly overwhelmed and anxious. For example, I coach founders and CEOs, who are usually, "Go, go, go, go!"

When you get busy, and your calendar gets blocked out, the No-Input Tuesday will be the first thing you want to ignore. But you've got to protect it like it's the Holy Grail because that is where the magic happens.

I've now got better at respecting the importance of 'being' time, and I go on walks every afternoon. I often stop computer work at about two and use the afternoons to think and be creative, but it's been the greatest gift. I love it.

Iain: Fantastic, I so believe that, and people won't get it until they start doing it.

But that focus, constantly being focused and do, do, do, is just a summary of 'the left hemisphere is now in control,' and nothing creative will happen. *Nothing.* You're just ensuring that nothing good is now going to come of this, so if you really want to fail badly, then just, *"Go for it, man!"*

What you need is to have controlled times of unfocus.

And for most people, the only moment in the day is when they're in the shower because you have to close your eyes, and you can't do anything.

So why is it that so many people's "Aha!" moments happen in the shower?

If you want a left hemisphere bullet point, "have more showers!" Haha.

Duncan: Haha.

Iain: But to be very serious, in what I'm writing, I've spent a lot of time reviewing how people make their breakthroughs and how good people's judgments are, and it's astonishing how much better it is when they're not fussing over it and trying to *make it happen*. It's usually when they're looking somewhere else, and then [click] it happens. And *then*, the drudgery of, "Well, I know that's right, but how am I going to justify it?" And then, they eventually find a way of doing so.

But the insight doesn't come by trying.

And life, what makes life fulfilling is the constant "Aha" moments, the moments of insight.

"A mind all logic is like a knife all blade.
It makes the hand bleed that uses it."

RABINDRANATH TAGORE

"Elite performers have something in common: They're really good at taking breaks."

DANIEL H. PINK

RUPERT SHELDRAKE, PHD

Former Dean and Director of Studies
in Biochemistry and Cell Biology
at Cambridge University, bestselling author
of *The Science Delusion.*

*In the West, we've popularized the idea of the individual,
independence, the lone cowboy. I wanted to understand
why and whether this was helping or hindering our
well-being.*

Atomized Individualism

Duncan: What do you mean by atomized individualism?

Rupert: It's a peculiar theory of society that grew up in the 17th century.

All traditional societies take it for granted that society is a unit; we're part of something bigger than ourselves. Without our families, we wouldn't survive, especially as babies. Without the larger society protecting and nurturing us, we wouldn't be here. All societies have moralities based on fitting in with others and cooperating.

And this is not just true of people; it's a basic biological fact.

Animal societies, packs of wolves, flocks of birds, ant and termite colonies, bees and wasps, all these social insects, all work for the good of a whole; it's not a matter of doing their own things. An ant isolated from its colony wouldn't survive very long, nor would a bee, a wasp, or a wolf.

But in the 17th century, Thomas Hobbs, one of the founders of modern science, put forward the idea of atomism in science.

He took up an old Greek idea that nature is made up of ultimate units of matter – atoms – that are separate and that society is made up of basic atoms, namely individuals.

And instead of seeing society as coming first and individuals being part of society, he saw individuals as coming first, with free will, free choice, and selfish desires. And society is imposing order on individuals.

But humans have never been isolated individuals.

Our ancestors were highly social, all tribal cultures, hunter-gatherers, were intensely social, and we're descended from apes, which are incredibly social: chimpanzees, bonobos, gorillas, monkeys, and their ancestors are intensely social animals.

There are more individualistic animals like snakes, crocodiles, and so on; reptiles, on the whole, are less social, but birds and mammals, most species are very social.

Anyway, the idea of Hobbs was that we're essentially individuals, free individuals, with free choice, and this gave rise to the philosophy of individualism that has so dominated the West.

It's all about me!

And society is something I have to live with or put up with, and it's annoying because it can restrain my freedom of choice and doing what I want.

This is entirely different from the attitude you find in India; I lived in India for seven years. I traveled and lived in Malaysia for a year. I've traveled in Sri Lanka several times. In Asian cultures, for most people, their family comes first and their social group – it's an entirely different mentality. They're usually rather appalled by the way in the West. "It's all about me," people move away from their family and have very little to do with them; when their parents get old, they're sent off to an old people's home, and the state's meant to look after them.

This way of living has developed in the West under this philosophy of extreme individualism. Which reaches its peak in the United States and probably reaches its highest pinnacle in Donald Trump. He represents the utmost in "me, me, me" individualism. That's why he strikes a chord with some Americans because they see him as an embodiment of this ultimate individualistic culture.

But the fact is that we're all completely dependent on other people, and it's an illusion to think that there's this individual atomistic society.

Yet, by behaving as if it's true, what happens is that traditional family bonds are dissolved, traditional social bonds are dissolved, traditional religious bonds are dissolved.

The fragmentation of families and the fragmentation of society leads to isolated people.

Huge numbers of people live alone now.

Many scientific studies show that lonely and isolated people get depressed more easily, their immune system doesn't work so well, and they're more prone to disease and infection. They're, generally speaking, much less happy because we're social animals; it's our nature to be social. The worst punishment that most governments can think of is putting people in solitary confinement.

So, unfortunately, we've got a social and political ideology that emphasizes individualism in the name of freedom.

And it's true, we're freer if we don't have to think about other people, but it's a significant limitation on the way we can live and the happiness that we can experience.

And, of course, depression is now the endemic disease of Western societies.

The Opposite of Gratefulness Is Feeling Entitled

Rupert: There's now a lot of evidence that grateful people are happier. And some critics said of this research, "Well, of course, they're grateful because they're happier." Well, it turns out they're happier because they're grateful.

Gratitude has measurable effects on people's happiness. All traditional cultures have ways of giving thanks, for example, before meals in the Christian tradition or the Jewish tradition.

The opposite of gratefulness is taking things for granted or feeling entitled and complaining if things aren't exactly as one might want them to be.

Grateful people are generally happier and more popular. Ungrateful people are generally unhappier and less popular.

FRED BRANSON

Co-Founder of Amantani, an award-winning
nonprofit that defends the rights
of indigenous children and young people
in the Peruvian Andes.

*Success. Happiness. Progress. Concepts like these are
relative. I wanted to speak to Fred about this.*

Progress?

Duncan: We often assume in the Westernized modern world
that we've got it 'right,' and this is how life should be, but you
could easily argue that many traditional communities have
a much better grasp and understanding of life.

Fred: Two sayings come to mind, one from the Quechua culture.
There's no word for 'poverty' in the Quechua language as we
understand it; there's no concept of poverty in that sense.

In their understanding of poverty, the poorest person would be
the person with the fewest people around them.

So essentially, poverty, for them, is loneliness.

And the other one that springs to mind. You're talking about
learning from traditions and ancient cultures, and I guess some
people would question if there's any merit in that and what
there is to learn?

In our fight for progress, we often think that the next generation knows more than the generation that preceded it.

However, I've spoken to some communities in Peru that believe each generation knows less than the one before it, which I loved as a concept of progress.

IDRIZ ZOGAJ

Five-time champion of Sweden's Best Memory, captained the Swedish national team to a Memory World Championship gold medal, founder of the Swedish Memory Association.

A few years ago, I became interested in the feats of memory athletes. I had no desire to become one, but I found the field fascinating. When you witness the 'impossible' repeated consistently, it forces you to recalibrate your beliefs. Idriz was the first Swedish person to memorize more than a thousand binary numbers (ones and zeroes) in thirty minutes. He was the first Swede to memorize an entire deck of cards in five minutes, then four minutes, then three. The athletes that compete do not have abilities reserved only for a special few. They are regular men and women who have trained their brains. And year after year, the records keep on falling. In 2019, Ryu Song I memorized 7485 binary digits. We are capable of so much more than we realize.

You Decide

Duncan: What's one thing all our listeners can do today that will positively affect their lives?

Idriz: Decide that *I am in control of my memory*, just as *I am in control of my body*. *You decide* that I have a good memory and I can put things in my memory. If you decide, *Okay, from today I'm going to remember better*, immediately, even without knowing anything about memory techniques, you will instantly raise your level.

Duncan: You've got to listen to the words you're saying. "I'm crap at languages," "I can't learn anything," "I'm no good at…" then okay, sure, that becomes your reality.

Idriz: Exactly.

THE STORIES WE TELL

I'm nineteen, traveling in South America with my girlfriend and staying in a hostel. I have never had a single hangover in my life, I have no idea why, but I don't get them.

One evening, we are drinking, and I decide that I want to have one of these mysterious things that everyone always complains about. I want to feel like shit tomorrow. I want to feel sorry for myself. I want to be in the hangover club!

This happens. The next day, I felt disgusting. Sadly, it isn't just the next day; every time I have anything to drink for the next three or four weeks, I feel terrible.

I'm not a massive fan of my new life skill. I never used to get hangovers, and I don't intend to keep them going forward, so I decide, "When I drink, I feel fine the next day." That was fifteen years ago, and when I drink, I feel fine the next day.

I have a terrible sense of direction. My day-to-day existence is a constant reminder of how bad my bearings are. If I'm walking down a street and decide to pop into a shop, upon leaving that building, I'll usually spend a few minutes walking back in the same direction I've just come from before it dawns on me what I've done, and I have to turn around again.

I've just passed my driver's test, and I'm now allowed to drive independently. I've lived in the same house for my entire life, and I'm now all grown up, self-reliant, and free to come and go as I like. I get into the car, turn the engine on, and put the gear stick into first gear. I then sit in our driveway for fifteen minutes, trying to determine if it's a left turn or a right to our local village.

"I have a terrible sense of direction." This is another story. I believe it and reinforce it, so it becomes an ingrained part of my identity. But like any story, it can be changed. My new story is, "I have a great sense of direction," and my life reflects this belief. Now it truly is good.

However, the example that I think about the most is this one. I've been seeing a girl for a while, we get on well, but we are not boyfriend and girlfriend. I think she's incredible, but I don't want to be in a relationship, so I'm upfront about this. After some months, she tells me that the way things are, is no longer working for her; she doesn't know if she's coming or going. Even though I care for her and we get on so well, I don't have strong feelings, so we decide to stop seeing each other. A few weeks pass. I realize I never even gave it a chance. I told myself a story, "I don't want to be in a relationship," and that was that.

I talk to her and say that I want to give things a proper go if she's still interested. I have felt detached, slightly distant, and had no real feelings for nine months, but when I see her the next day, I am overwhelmed with love for her.

I don't know how or why? What has changed? She hasn't changed. She is the beautiful, creative, funny girl she has always been. All that has changed is my story. My new story is "I want to be with her."

Your life is a reflection of the stories you believe. Beliefs are stories. If your story is *life is hard,* or *I'm unlucky in love,* or fill in the blank… Then your life will reflect that.

What stories are you telling yourself?

LYNNE MCTAGGART

Award-winning journalist, co-founder and editor of *What Doctors Don't Tell You*, bestselling author of *The Bond: The Power of Connection*.

The term 'quantum physics' is fun to say. It sounds intelligent. I would sometimes slip it into sentences even though I had no idea what it meant. Was it even relevant to well-being? I needed to track down someone who did understand it.

An Endless Game of Tennis

Lynne: First of all, I want to put on the table that what I really hate is unsupported woo woo! I really do. I have a background as an investigative reporter; that's where I came from and started my life, so that desire to have evidence for things has never left me.

When we talk about 'we're all one,' on a quantum level, we are all one because we're made up of subatomic particles. Subatomic particles aren't individual entities like a billiard ball, as described in high school physics. They are vibrating packets of energy that trade energy with other vibrating packets of energy all the time, like an endless game of tennis.

So if you factor in all of those little tennis games going on, there is an unbelievable, unfathomable amount of energy being traded in empty space.

First of all, that creates a giant energy field.

There are two intriguing things about subatomic particles.

1) They have an infinite capacity for information.

2) They go on forever.

And so, if you think of this mothership of quantum field that's sitting out there in empty space like some super-charged backdrop, it's a memory bank for everything that ever was, and we are part of that. We essentially have access to everything in the universe and each other. So we are all connected on a quantum level.

And secondly, on the connection between people, scientists have discovered that we're a lot less individual than we think we are. There are neurons in our head – mirror neurons – that when we see someone else perform an action or have an emotion, the same neurons in us fire. Like we were experiencing that emotion, we were performing that action.

So we've been designed to have this so that we can empathize with other people.

But what that essentially means is that our brains, our minds, what we're dealing with all the time is a complex mix of our own thoughts and everybody else's thoughts.

Altruism Is Like a Bulletproof Vest

Lynne: I've looked at the science of altruism, and altruism is like a bulletproof vest.

Whenever there's an altruistic thing, the givers do better than the receivers.

For instance, there's a study on depression. A scientist who was also a priest – he was a psychologist and priest – wanted to see if praying for people with depression would help them because most prayer is for physical, not mental illness. So he got a group of four hundred people diagnosed with clinical depression. He divided them into two groups and had one half be the senders/ the prayers, and the other ones being the prayed for, and he measured what happened to them afterward very scientifically.

And he found that the people being prayed for did well.

But the people doing the praying did even better. They were far less depressed.

And if you look at all the science of altruism, you see the same thing. People who give, whatever they give, if there's some giving in any capacity, the givers live longer and are healthier. If they have a condition and they're helping someone else with that condition, they do better than the recipient.

What's Wrong with Self-Help? The Self.

Lynne: A guy called West was a Vietnam vet, and he was supposed to go to college and get a science degree. He had a whole life plan, and it got derailed because he received a low lottery number for the Vietnam War, which meant you go off to war, so he was part of that last year, and it was incredibly traumatic for him. He was very depressed by it, and his life continued down in an ever-lowering spiral. He found the love of his life in the late nineties, and she lived for a few years, and then she died of cancer, and he had enormous bills, had to sell his house to pay the bills back. It was shocking and awful.

He was part of a small Power of Eight group (eight people in a group who carry out an intention for each other) that I assembled about two months ago, and he was a sender; he was not even a receiver. And he said he had this almost epiphany of rejuvenation like suddenly the grass was looking greener, and the flowers were smelling sweeter, and he had got to the point in his life of *What's the use?* He's in his mid-sixties; life had been so crap for him. And suddenly, he had all this rejuvenation to get back and do things and all kinds of things. And that has happened over and over and over again. The people doing the sending have physical healings, mental healings, they have some rejuvenation like this, where life makes sense, has a purpose, they find their life's purpose.

I have thought a lot about this and about some of the dangerous elements of the self-help movement because it's all that focus on the self!

Duncan: Yeah. Me, me, me.

Lynne: That could be toxic.

The Brainwave Activity of Good Intentions

Lynne: Life University, the largest chiropractor university, offered me their psychology department to do a series of studies, and the first one's been done already. We looked at the brainwave activity of the senders of good intentions – the senders, not the receivers – and we found that there was this kind of global quieting of the brain, of the part:

1) The parietal lobes. Which makes us feel separate like this is where we end [pointing to her body] and the rest of the universe begins [pointing outside her body].

2) The frontal lobes. And they're very much involved in, again, separation, a sense of me [pointing to her body] and not me [pointing outside], but also doubt, worry, all those negative things. That stuff was all turned way down.

Those brainwaves were a signature almost identical to the work of Andrew Newberg, who's done a lot of brainwave studies of Sufi masters and Buddhist monks in ecstatic prayer.

But what was so interesting about our situation is that they weren't looking at people who required years of disciplined practice or who needed hours of priming to get into that state. These were total novices who'd had a fifteen-minute video from me explaining how to do this, and all they needed was a group, and they had some fast-track to an ecstatic state of mind.

GREGG BRADEN

Transformational leader, invited to speak to the
United Nations and the U.S. military, bestselling
author of *The Science of Self-Empowerment:
Awakening the New Human Story.*

*I always enjoy speaking with holistic thinkers, individuals
who can zoom out and appreciate the interplay of
different systems. There are so many things we don't
know. There are so many future discoveries, at present,
still invisible to us. I think it's important to celebrate and
encourage the cross-pollination of ideas. Gregg is a big
picture thinker, so I was keen to hear what he had to say.*

Who Are We?

Gregg: You and I, Duncan, and our listeners are steeped in a scientific story about ourselves that is based on false information. We have been taught that the world, nature, the fundamental rule of nature is competition and conflict. This is the world we live in. Our economic system is based upon this; our corporate systems are based upon this. Our medical model is based upon this. The way we share food, medicine, water, and vital resources is based upon this conscious and subconscious thinking.

If you ask a scientist, "Who are we?" a scientist to answer that question will say, "I must first answer six sub-questions, six fundamental sub-questions." So here's what a scientist will ask, beginning with a very fundamental question:

1) What is the origin of life – where does life come from in general?

2) Where does human life come from?

3) What is our relationship to our bodies?

4) What is our relationship to the world beyond our bodies?

5) What is our relationship to the past?

6) What is the fundamental rule of nature?

For a hundred and fifty years, we in the Western world have been steeped in a story that answers those questions in a way we now know is false, and it's based upon separation, competition, and conflict.

We've been told the origin of life is completely random.

The origin of human life is completely random; evolution is our story.

We've been told that we're essentially powerless when it comes to influencing the healing of our bodies.

We have been told that we're essentially powerless when it comes to influencing the events of the world around us.

Civilization, we're told that it began five thousand years ago. We are the pinnacle of sophistication, the most advanced that this planet has ever seen.

And number six, the fundamental rule of nature since the 1850s, we've been told that nature is based on survival of the strongest; those are the exact words, later interpreted as survival of the fittest, but in Charles Darwin's book, survival of the strongest, competition, and conflict.

Peer-reviewed science has overturned every single one of those.

And now we know when we ask, "Who are we?"

The origin of life? It's not random.

The origin of human life? The new DNA shows us that there are intentional changes, splicing of chromosomes in our bodies that cannot be accounted for through evolution alone. It is not a random process.

When it comes to our bodies? We're deeply connected. Thoughts, feelings, emotions, and beliefs change the chemistry in our bodies. And we get to choose the emotions that change the chemistry.

When it comes to the world beyond our bodies? Quantum physics now tells us there's no controversy that we are connected. That is accepted in quantum physics now. We are connected to one another and our world.

Here's the controversy, to *what degree* are we connected? How *much* influence do we have in the world? That's where scientists are struggling right now, but they acknowledge that we are connected.

Civilization? When it comes to civilization, what we know now is that new archaeological discoveries have pushed the dates for advanced technological civilizations back into the last ice age – over twice as old as what we're teaching our kids in school. We've been on this planet for a long time, and we know things from the past that can benefit us today; that's the value of looking at it.

And last but not least, the best science of the twenty-first century is now telling us that nature is based upon a model of cooperation and what biologists call *mutual aid*.

And it doesn't deny that competition happens; we've all seen it.

But here's the thing: the more competition and the more conflict we see in the world around us, that tells us how far we have strayed from the truest, most fundamental law of nature that we are not honoring:

We're going against the flow.

We're fighting the tide.

DEBRA PONEMAN

Transformational leader and bestselling author who taught many of today's household names such as Deepak Chopra.

In the 1980s, Debra Poneman founded Yes to Success Seminars. She brought into the mainstream radical ideas like "your thoughts create your reality." Within a few years, her seminars were being taught globally, all before the days of the internet. Many of her students went on to become New York Times bestsellers and household names.

Building Relationship Capital

Debra: When my son was fifteen, he started a business. Do you know this?

Duncan: No.

Debra: He started a business where he recruited high school basketball players for college coaches. He made the A-team in basketball in his freshman year in high school, and he never got any playing time, but he still had to go to all of the games – the freshman, JV, varsity games, and he noticed that he had an eye for talent. So he started a website, and he became the go-to person at fifteen years old for the biggest coaches in college basketball.

We'd be at dinner; he'd say, "Got to go. Bill Carmody's on the phone."

I mean, really? These are massive names! There was a full-page article in Sports Illustrated about him when he was sixteen: 'Why College Hoops Coaches Seek the Advice of a Sixteen-Year-Old Scout.'

But here's the point: he did it for free because he saw these kids in the hood who didn't have anybody advocating for them, not the Division I but the Division II kids. He started putting on showcases for them so college hoops coaches could come and see these Division II kids.

And he's been doing it ever since. He just had one a couple of weeks ago. There were two hundred and fifty kids and a hundred and twenty college coaches representing ninety-eight schools. And between when he started, and now, he's gotten over $25 million in college scholarships for his kids, and he doesn't take a penny because he is all about giving; he is all about serving.

And now he's just become an official NBA agent, so he'll make a ton of money, and *everybody* wants to help him, everybody wants to give him contacts, everybody wants to connect him because he's getting payback. He didn't do it for the payback. But when you do that selfless service, when you serve from your heart, when you do what your heart prompts even though it doesn't seem like it's making any money...

Worried for him, I would say, "Daniel, you're not making any money."

He'd say, "Mum, I'm building relationship capital."

And he did.

"When takers win, there's usually someone else who loses. Research shows that people tend to envy successful takers and look for ways to knock them down a notch. In contrast, when givers win, people are rooting for them and supporting them, rather than gunning for them. Givers succeed in a way that creates a ripple effect, enhancing the success of people around them."

ADAM GRANT, PHD

STEVE FARBER

Business and leadership expert, President
of Extreme Leadership Inc., bestselling
author of *Greater Than Yourself: The Ultimate
Lesson of True Leadership*.

*I had learned how being kind, loving, and altruistic
makes us feel happier. But how does love apply to
business? There were two reasons why I needed to speak
with Steve Farber. The first is that Steve is one of the
top leadership experts in the world. The second reason
is that he looks like Robert De Niro. So I can now lie
and say I've also interviewed him.*

The Greatest Leaders

Steve: Somehow, we have come to believe that business is a zero-sum game, that my success has to be predicated on you not being as successful as I am, or even worse, maybe even on your failure. This whole idea of dog eat dog, get ahead, get ahead by crushing somebody else's head, climbing the proverbial corporate ladder on the backs of everybody else. But when you look at it, that's not the way it works.

I've been doing this kind of work for a long time. By *this kind of work*, I mean cultivating great leadership in the business world, been doing it for twenty-five-plus years, and so this is not ideology, and it's not idealism; it's based on a simple observation.

The greatest leaders that I've met are the ones that don't focus the attention on their own greatness. They don't shine the spotlight on themselves; they don't try to grab all the credit. Instead, they focus their efforts on making others greater than themselves. So it creates a bit of a paradox.

The greatest leaders become the greatest leaders by making others greater than themselves.

And they understand that it's not a zero-sum game. It's not that for every winner, there's a loser. It's that we can all help each other, and I'm going to be the example of that as a leader; I'm going to build my credibility and establish my track record based on how many superstars I've helped to create by virtue of their working with me, for me, around me, whatever it is. So it's this investment in other people.

Man, I mean, can you imagine, can you imagine if that were the norm? Can you imagine if that's just how we believed we should do things? How different not just business would be, but everything.

Love Is Damn Good Business

Steve: Love is at the very foundation of what great leadership is, and it's just damn good business. Love is good business. Does that sound weird to you?

Duncan: It doesn't, maybe because I've been having these conversations. It now seems obvious – of course, love is good business – but I could perhaps imagine a few years ago where that would seem like a foreign, alien concept. Love? Business? What?

Steve: I'm not exaggerating when I say this, and I'm not saying it to toot my own horn. But over the last two and a half decades,

I have worked with literally every kind of industry you can imagine. Worked directly with, spoken to, or had exposure to every type of business you can imagine. So I have this really broad perspective on things, and it's become easy for me to see what the universal elements are.

And when I look at the big picture, it doesn't matter what the business is. It doesn't matter what the industry is. It doesn't matter what part of the planet people are on; certain things emerge as being universally true. So no matter where I go, no matter what business I'm involved in, I see that love is the principle that makes great leaders great.

If you want happiness for an hour,
take a nap.
If you want happiness for a day,
go fishing.
If you want happiness for a month,
get married.
If you want happiness for a year,
inherit a fortune.
If you want happiness for a lifetime,
help somebody else.

CHINESE PROVERB

"I slept and dreamt that life was joy. I awoke and saw that life was service. I acted and behold, service was joy."

RABINDRANATH TAGORE

ONE THING AT A TIME

One of the most impactful changes in my life over the last four or five years has been adopting the mentality of *one thing at a time*.

When I'm eating, I'm eating.

When I'm watching a film, I'm only watching a film.

If I'm having a conversation with someone, that is the only thing I'm doing.

I used to regularly eat food in front of the TV while talking and glancing at my phone. Everything was getting a fraction of my watered-down attention.

Since embracing the idea of one thing at a time and actually sticking to it, routine tasks have become more fun, simple meals and flavors taste more delicious, and conversations and spending time with people is richer and more enjoyable.

Life is far more colorful.

It feels like choosing between an old, grainy, pixelated screen versus one with high-definition.

TIM KASSER, PHD

Emeritus Professor of Psychology, featured expert
in the documentaries *Happy* and *The True Cost*,
author of *The High Price of Materialism*.

*What type of goals increase happiness? What type of
goals decrease happiness? How do our values affect our
well-being? Tim Kasser is the world's leading authority
on the psychology of materialism and consumer culture.*

Extrinsic Goals vs. Intrinsic Goals

Duncan: Extrinsic materialistic goals and intrinsic goals. What is the difference between those two?

Tim: Values and goals are the things we're striving for in life, the things that we find important, the stuff we're trying to make happen. And they help us decide what to do in life, what behaviors to engage in, how we feel about different political candidates or different kinds of clothes or whatever it might be.

The work that we've been doing for more than twenty years now has made a distinction about the content of people's values and goals. We distinguish between what we call extrinsic materialistic goals and intrinsic goals.

The materialistic extrinsic goals are the ones that are by and large encouraged by consumer culture. They are things like trying to have a lot of money, or the right image, trying to be popular and high status. And we call those extrinsic goals because they're focused on external rewards. They're focused on getting money, getting the gold star in school, having other people say, "Oh, don't you look great," or whatever.

Then we contrast those with intrinsic goals, and intrinsic goals are goals that are inherently satisfying to pursue. They're goals like your own personal growth or connecting with the community, or having close interpersonal relationships. And there's a lot of different research that shows there's a fundamental tension between these intrinsic and extrinsic goals and that they operate in opposition to each other.

What we've found over and over, in a couple of hundred studies, researchers have demonstrated that when people prioritize materialistic values for money, image, and status, they report that they're less happy. They're less satisfied with their lives, feel less vital, and experience fewer positive emotions like joy and contentment. They're also more depressed, anxious, and more likely to use substances like alcohol, cigarettes, etc.

Think of Your Values as a Pie

Duncan: It's like a seesaw. If you focus on materialistic things, then the intrinsic things have to give?

Tim: Yeah, that's right. Another analogy I use a lot is to think about all your values as being a big pie, and each slice of the pie is a different value. So you have a spirituality slice, a family slice, a hedonism slice, a materialism slice, and everybody's got a slice of each.

As one piece of the pie gets bigger, some other pieces have to get smaller. And what the research demonstrates, and this is the seesaw effect, is that it's not random which values will get smaller as materialistic values get bigger. It's not a random thing.

As materialism becomes more and more important, you're going to see image and popularity become more important, and you're going to see the intrinsic values shrink.

But the opposite is also true. As people focus more and more on those intrinsic values, for their growth, for connections to family and community, as that slice gets bigger and bigger, the materialistic slice tends to shrink.

Duncan: If you know you are focusing on the wrong things, that's scary. But like you said, on the flip side, we're in control. We can choose to focus on those intrinsic things. I think that's an empowering thought.

Tim: Yeah, I think it is too, and I want to emphasize that all of us have all of the values. I know that I'm materialistic some days, and I've been studying its problems for twenty-something years. But the question becomes, what do you do when those materialistic values get activated in you – how do you behave?

And how do you organize your whole life to decrease how much time you spend in that part of your value system? And increase how much time you're spending in the intrinsic part of your value system?

JOEL FOTINOS

Businessman, Vice-President at St. Martin's Press, former Vice-President at Tarcher/Penguin, author of *My Life Contract*.

I love books. An author might spend thirty years researching a topic; within a few hours, we have the opportunity to absorb that wisdom. This is also why I love interviewing people. I wanted to speak with Joel because he sits in various camps. Business, spirituality, human potential. He has been studying transformation for decades.

Why Are You Here?

Joel: One simple question: why are you here? The very thing we're so afraid of, if we say, why are you here? And begin a relationship with it; it transforms. We don't have to run from it anymore. We can stop and be empowered by it rather than be diminished by it. It's a way of going through life where we are not ruled by fear.

I noticed there was a period a few years ago when I was watching a lot of horror movies like *Friday the 13*th, *I Know What You Did Last Summer* and *Halloween*. I was watching them, but I wasn't even sure why I was watching them, and I thought, *what is it in these movies that is speaking to me right now?*

And one thing I noticed in those movies is that, for the first two-thirds of the film, all the people are scared to death of the thing that's trying to kill them, so they're running from that thing, and they're trying to hide. And the thing that they're trying to hide from *always* shows up. It's always right behind them or right behind the door.

But in every single one of those movies, a point happens where they think, *I can't live this way anymore*, and they turn around. And instead of being hunted by the thing they're afraid of, they start trying to hunt and find it, whether it's Freddie or the Bogeyman. And the minute they turn around and try to find the thing that has been finding them, it shifts the whole movie, and of course, they end up winning at the end of the film.

And I thought *that's what this is*. We are so afraid of certain things in our lives, and when we're afraid of them, it's like they are chasing us; they are always right where we are.

And we think we've escaped them using maybe alcohol or shopping or – for me – credit cards or sex or this or that or watching TV or spending hours on the computer. And we think we've got a handle on it, yet it always pops up, right there, and it's always there.

So when we get active and turn around and say, "No, you're not going to hunt me anymore. I'm now going to look for you," then suddenly we are not ruled by it. We are taking control of our life and are empowered.

It always changes things.

Why are you here?

Energy Follows Action

Duncan: Energy follows action.

Why is just starting so important? Even if we have no idea what we are doing.

Joel: Because it's the formula for life, and I was one of those people who, for many years, tried to live the other way. I kept saying to myself, "I will do better as soon as I have more money," "I will be more charitable as soon as I pay off my debt," and "I will do *this* as soon as *that* happens." And what ended up happening is that nothing happened. I stayed stuck. I kept not moving, and then I recognized that what I wanted to happen couldn't happen until I was actually in action. So I had to begin by taking action. As soon as I took action, the whole energy of the situation changed completely.

KAMAL RAVIKANT

Entrepreneur, investor, bestselling author
of *Love Yourself Like Your Life
Depends on It.*

*I was watching a talk on YouTube by a venture capitalist.
The man was a well-known figure in the Silicon Valley
startup scene. But the topic wasn't about success or
making money. Instead, he spoke about the failure of
a company he'd spent more than a decade nurturing.
He described the humiliation and depression he felt
and the self-love required to get up from that point.
This isn't what we're speaking about below, but it's
why I was curious to learn more about what Kamal
had to say.*

Modeling Success

Kamal: I saw this amazing talk with Warren Buffett the other
night, and he was talking to these MBA students. He said, "If
I was to tell you, pick one person out of here, out of your peer
group, and you're guaranteed ten percent of their earnings for
their whole life, who would you pick?" And he said, "I bet you,
you won't pick the one with the highest grades." This is Warren
Buffett; he's sharp, he's right. You'll pick a person with certain
qualities and attributes. So ask yourself, who's that person you're
going to pick and why? What are those attributes that are mak-

ing you choose them? Then take those attributes and start to work on having them yourself.

That's such a great exercise because immediately, what is it that you look up to? And then you work to become, to have those attributes yourself. When he was sixteen, Benjamin Franklin used to do this himself – what virtues did he want to develop?

All these things are learned, they're patterns, and they're conditioned. We can practice them and become them.

This thing [pointing to his brain] is very plastic – able to change and grow – and there's a lot of freedom in that.

> **Note**: *Success leaves clues.*
>
> *But also, happiness leaves clues.*
>
> *The story above is about business, but the same principle applies to life. How can we identify qualities and attributes that we admire and work on developing those ourselves?*
>
> *This is not to be confused with trying to be someone else, losing your identity, or being inauthentic.*
>
> *If I became a father for the first time, I might think, who is a great parent, in my opinion? Why do I think that? Maybe it's because they are patient, they allow their kids to make mistakes and grow, are loving, and are present. I can then develop these attributes and become the parent I want to be. I'm not losing my identity and trying to be that person.*
>
> *It's the same with this book. I'm sharing advice from the best happiness experts in the world. If you want to be happy, here are habits that you should practice.*
>
> *You're still you. You're still authentic. You've just identified an area – happiness – that you want to grow in.*

MICHAEL SHERMER, PHD

Founder/publisher of *Skeptic* magazine,
Presidential Fellow at Chapman University,
bestselling author of *The Believing Brain*.

*How can we avoid some common pitfalls that prevent
clear reasoning? How can we make better decisions?
I wanted to speak with Michael about how to think.*

The Moment You Comprehend an Idea, You Believe It

Duncan: Belief and believing in things is our natural state. We
want to believe in things.

Michael: Yeah, so the default action of the brain is the moment
you comprehend an idea, you believe it, it must be true, or else
why would you be comprehending it?

So skepticism is an additional cognitive load, another step
you have to take to say, "Now that I comprehend it, I wonder
if it's true? I got the claim, but is the claim true?" That takes
another step. And this is why skepticism does not come naturally; it feels uncomfortable, it feels like a load of work, like,
"Ohh, it would just be so much easier to believe this rather than
having to comprehend it and *then* go a step further and play
the devil's advocate to your brain and say, 'Wait a minute, wait
a minute, Shermer, *maybe,* I'd like it to be this way, but *maybe*
it isn't that way?'"

I was having a discussion with Dan Dennett yesterday about Snowden. At first, I didn't like what Snowden did with the Wikileaks thing. Then I saw him at the TED conference, calling in from a remote location in Moscow. He came across as totally, completely honest, full of integrity, and a freedom lover. I'm a big freedom lover guy, big libertarian, and I was like, "Yes! Yes! Government overreach, the NSA, no good! I love this guy! *I love this guy!*"

But this is just reinforcing what I want to be true.

And then I'm reading this article the other day in *The Wall Street Journal* about maybe he wasn't the good guy all of a sudden. I'm like, "Oh no," and I don't like reading that; I have to force myself because I'd rather have things be true the way *I want them* to be true.

We Are Pattern Seekers

Duncan: Humans are pattern seekers; this has been beneficial for us, for example, when spotting risks. You can hear a distant rustle. Is that just the wind, or is it maybe a saber-toothed tiger ready to pounce at you? So this is a good thing; we spot patterns, which has helped us evolutionarily. But it's also problematic.

Michael: Well, at least to things like conspiracy thinking, where you think, *there's a pattern, maybe there's an even deeper pattern?*

The Illuminati!

There are twelve guys in London smoking cigars and drinking whiskey and deciding the economies of the world and the political organizations of the world!

Our brains naturally go to that, but as you said, finding patterns is good. Is global warming real, or isn't it? Are we causing it or not? That's a pattern. And in principle, science should be able to answer that question. When did the universe begin? Is it expanding forever, or is it going to collapse? That's a pattern, and we can figure it out.

Unfortunately, the default position is to believe it the moment you put the pattern together; *A is connected to B, C, and D.* You think it must be real. *Princess Diana was murdered by the royal family.* Then you start looking for evidence to fit it when going through the daily newspaper or wherever, *Oooo look, look, look what I just found! There must be some connection!*

That's patternicity.

But that's not good because our brains are then acting more like lawyers, marshaling evidence in support of your client – in this case, your belief. Rather than being the devil's advocate and saying, "Wait a minute, what would it take to falsify my belief? I want this to be true. I think this is true. Now, what would it take for me to change my mind?"

That's a much, much harder thing to do. It's hard to even think of examples that don't fit. And this is why we need to force ourselves to read newspapers or magazines and opinions that we don't like. I do this. I'm a libertarian, I can find fault with both liberals and conservatives, but I force myself to listen to people I disagree with just so I can think, *Well, wait a minute, Shermer, maybe, maybe I'm wrong about this?* So it forces me to change my mind.

Like on gun control, I changed my mind. The death penalty, I changed my mind. I used to be for it in support of the victim's families. But then I rationally analyzed it by people that are critical of the death penalty, who I normally don't like; I don't agree with them. They're uber-liberal, California, bla bla bla, and it's like, "No, you know what, I think they're right," and I changed my mind.

It's hard to do. I'm not saying I'm anything special. I'm like everybody else – I'd rather just blindly go on believing what I want to be true.

"Giving people more control over what they do
and how they do it increases their happiness,
engagement, and sense of fulfillment."

CAL NEWPORT, PHD

"The evidence shows people who are unemployed feel even worse than people in meaningless jobs. The primary way in which meaningless work causes depression is through a lack of control – and unemployed people have even *less* control over their lives. They have no financial resources, no social status, and no choices about their lives."

JOHANN HARI

NICK JANKEL

Futurist, creator of Bio-Transformation Theory, has taught at Oxford University, London Business School, and Yale. Author of *Switch On.*

Nick is an interdisciplinary thinker. He has a great depth and breadth of knowledge: medicine, regeneration, A.I., social innovation, ancient wisdom, and the science of transformation.

No Awards Will Ever Relieve That Feeling

Nick: One of the most important things I've ever learned is that trying to change things deeply held within us by changing things outside, literally, logically, can only fail.

If you've got a deep sense of lack of connection to your dad, your mum, nature, you feel let down by what you thought was God when you were seven, your siblings, whatever. If you feel any profound lack that is consistent and has been for many years, and it's inside. And you try and fill that up with sex, drugs, dancing, work, entrepreneurship, reputation, fame, fortune, anything outside you; it can never work, and that's addiction.

People say, "I'm not addicted." But I would say 99.9% of people are addicted to something, whether it's checking your Facebook to see if anyone's liked you today, whether it's rising at work, so you spend two more hours there than others. Whatever it is, we're all addicted to something, which is trying to fulfill this emptiness inside, this hole inside.

That hole is powerful because what it does is it starts driving a lot of your thoughts and behaviors out of a place of fear or lack or pain or suffering. Because one of the things we've learned in the last twenty years since I was at medical school is that we are fundamentally emotionally-driven beings.

So if our systems are being driven by emotion and we have a consistent emotion within us of lack, fear, or loss, then no matter how much we try and change the behaviors, there's still the emotion anchoring those behaviors in place.

If you are working really hard because you feel like you never got the respect from your folks or never felt seen by them, let's say you never felt seen by them, which is a big thing for many people. So you work really hard, and then you realize you can never work hard enough, you can never win employee of the month awards or even something grand like a TED Fellowship; nothing you ever win is ever going to relieve that feeling that people haven't seen you until you heal it inside.

And the thing is those people are no longer around, they could well be dead, or if not, they're probably just not in your life as much as they used to be. So there's no point in saying to your dad, who's sixty or whatever, "I never felt seen by you," and he goes, "Well, I see you." It doesn't make a difference; you still won't feel seen because the memories of not being seen are deep inside.

And an interesting thing about the brain is your pain memories, the ones that are really like, *Pwwwooh, this was a painful moment*, are much nearer your amygdala than other memories, so they're really ready to trigger you into a certain set of habits or patterns.

If you want to transform something, not just change a little bit but transform something profoundly anchored inside you, a way of relating to the world, let's say. One of my ones used to be that I always wanted to get to the next thing, so I was always very like, "Okay, what's the next thing, what's the next thing?" What I used to call a fast forward button in my life. That's another learned habit, a way of avoiding being in the moment because the moment's quite painful, so if I get to the next moment, I can get more excited about it.

So if I'm going to change that – yes, being aware of it, going to therapy is really helpful – but until I alter the emotional feeling of what it feels like to be in the moment, I'll always use that or another addiction or habit to get out of the moment.

And you have to do that work because no one else will do it for you. That's the great work of life, I think, is to do that work, to give yourself the love, attention, connection, and sense of self-purpose that you didn't get as a kid.

And when you do that and not just once – *I saw myself! I feel loved!* Okay, great, until the next time you're triggered into feeling sad or lonely or upset. Realize that that's just the beginning of the gate, open into the challenges of living a switched-on life in every moment, integrating it, embedding it, and embodying it. So that slowly, over time, you become a person whose natural response to life is collaboration, compassion, caring, purpose, all the things we know we want. It just becomes more and more natural. And I'm by no means "finished" on that process.

WHAT HAPPENED TO YOU? WHAT IS HAPPENING TO YOU?

Duncan: Shame is known to make people sick.

Even when they received medical care at the same point in their illness during the AIDS crisis, closeted gay men, on average, died two to three years earlier than openly gay men.

Johann Hari: This was the cause of depression and anxiety that I found hardest to learn about for personal reasons. To explain this, I have to tell you a story that's going to sound for a minute like I'm talking about some entirely different thing. But it led to a breakthrough in depression and anxiety, and I don't think you can understand that breakthrough if you don't understand how it was discovered.

In the mid-1980s, a doctor who I got to know called Dr. Vincent Felitti in San Diego was given quite a difficult task. Kaiser Permanente is one of the big not-for-profit medical providers in California, and they had this massive problem. There's a vast and growing obesity crisis. Everything they were trying, like, giving people nutritional advice and exercise programs, wasn't making much difference. So they gave Vincent a load of money, and they said, look, do blue skies research, figure out what the hell's going on here because we can't carry on like this.

So Dr. Felitti started to work with three hundred and fifty severely obese people, people who weighed in most cases more than four hundred pounds, so really, really obese, and people who'd tried everything and nothing was working. So this is like the last chance saloon.

And he starts to work with them, and he's just brainstorming ideas. One day he has what seems like a very dumb idea. He thought, what would happen if they just stopped eating? And we gave them nutritional supplements, so they didn't get scurvy or whatever – would they burn through the fat stores in their body until they got down to a normal weight? Obviously, with mega-intense medical supervision, they started to do this, and the crazy thing is, in one way, it worked.

I'll give you an example: a woman; I will call her Susan to protect her medical confidentiality. Susan had been more than four hundred pounds; she went down to a hundred and thirty-eight pounds. People are celebrating, calling Vincent a lifesaver, Susan's family is thanking God, and then something happens that no one anticipated. One day, Susan freaked out and fled and started gorging on fast food, and very quickly, she got back to not quite what she was, but a dangerous weight.

And Vincent called her in, and he said, "Susan, what happened?"

And she looked down and said, "I don't know, I don't know."

And he said, "Well, did anything happen that day? Tell me about that day that you cracked."

Something did happen that day that hadn't ever happened to Susan: a man hit on her. When she was very obese, men didn't hit on her. A colleague tried to sleep with her, not a sexual assault or anything, but hitting on her. It really frightened her.

And then, at a later session, Vincent said, "Susan, when did you start to put on weight?"

She said it was when she was ten.

He said, "Well, did anything happen when you were ten that didn't happen when you were eight, didn't happen when you were fourteen – why when you were ten?"

And she looked down and said, "Well, that's when my grandfather started to rape me."

When he interviewed them, it turned out that fifty-five percent of the people in the program had put on their weight in the aftermath of being sexually assaulted or abused.

Vincent was really puzzled by this – what's going on? He started to think that this thing that appears to be a pathology – and in one sense is obviously a pathology: obesity – actually had a deep, underlying reason; it was sexually protective.

Susan said to Vincent, "Overweight is overlooked, and that's what I need to be."

But this is quite a small study, so Vincent decided to do a much larger study, which led to this breakthrough in depression. So he got a load of funding from the CDC, the Center for Disease Control, one of the huge bodies in the U.S. that funds these things, the gold standard. Everyone who came to Kaiser Permanente in San Diego for a year for anything, whether headaches, broken leg, schizophrenia, anything, was given a questionnaire.

The first part of the questionnaire said, "Did any of these ten bad things happen to you when you were a kid," such as physical abuse, sexual abuse, neglect, etc. And then they were asked, "Have you had any of these ten problems as an adult," things like obesity, addiction. At the last minute, they added depression and suicide attempts.

When the CDC added up the results, they were just astonished. For every category of childhood trauma you experienced, you were radically more likely to become depressed and anxious.

If you'd had six of those categories, you were 3100% more likely to have attempted suicide as an adult. You don't get figures like that in epidemiology often; it's an extraordinary result.

And it goes to exactly what you're asking about, Duncan. It goes to shame; there's a reason we know that. When I went to go and see Vincent in San Diego the first time, I remember being angry, really enraged with him. I was like, *why am I so pissed off with this guy?*

When I was a child, I experienced some very extreme acts from an adult in my life. My mother had been very ill, my dad was in a different country, and I experienced these extreme acts. And I think I found the "depression is just caused by a chemical imbalance in the brain" theory so appealing because I didn't want to think about these things. I didn't want to believe that this individual had any power over me; I didn't want to consider it was playing out in my life now. Seeing Vincent meant I had to reintegrate these experiences into how I thought about my own depression, which was painful.

Everyone who filled in this questionnaire and said they'd experienced childhood trauma, the next time they went to the doctor, the doctor was told to say to the patient something like, "So, I see that when you were a child, you were sexually abused," or whatever it was, "I'm really sorry that happened to you, that should never have happened, would you like to talk about it?" And a significant minority said, "No, I don't want to talk about it," but most people did. Average conversation lasted five minutes, at the end of which it was randomized, and some of them were told, "We can refer you to a therapist if you'd like to."

What was fascinating is that five-minute conversation where an authority figure said, "I'm really sorry, that shouldn't have happened, this should never have happened to you," that alone led to a really significant fall in depression and anxiety. And the people referred to a therapist had a bigger fall.

And this is part of a broader body of evidence. Professor James Pennebaker has done excellent research on this, precisely about releasing shame. If you go through these things, you internalize a lot of shame for all sorts of complex reasons.

Dr. Robert Anda said a beautiful line to me. He said that when you see people behaving in ways that seem so strange, whether it's depression, anxiety, addiction, obesity, we need to stop asking, "What's wrong with you?" And start asking, "What happened to you?"

And I would say, in line with all the other research, "What is happening to you?"

IT HAS MEANING EVERY TIME

GABOR MATÉ, MD

"All of the diagnoses that you deal with – depression, anxiety, ADHD, bipolar illness, post-traumatic stress disorder, even psychosis, are significantly rooted in trauma. They are manifestations of trauma. Therefore, the diagnoses don't explain anything. The problem in the medical world is that we diagnose somebody and we think that is the explanation. He's behaving that way because he is psychotic. She's behaving that way because she has ADHD. Nobody has ADHD, nobody has psychosis – these are processes within the individual. It's not a thing that you have.

This is a process that expresses your life experience.

It has meaning in every single case."

KEVIN KELLY

Digital visionary, co-founder of *Wired* magazine, bestselling author of *The Inevitable: Understanding the 12 Technological Forces that Will Shape Our Future.*

Does being a long-term thinker affect our sense of satisfaction? It wasn't hard to think who I should speak to about this. New York Times bestselling author Kevin Kelly has the longest time frame of anyone I've ever met. He's championed projects that look ten thousand years into the future at the 'Long Now Foundation.' And he is behind visionary organizations such as the 'All Species Foundation,' a non-profit aimed at identifying and cataloging every living species on earth.

Short-Term Thinking vs. Long-Term Thinking

Duncan: Instant gratification.

You want a date? Swipe! You've got a date. You want a car? Click! It's outside. We want everything now, now, now! But making things better requires long-term thinking.

Kevin: It does. The advantage of long-term thinking is that it can give you more fulfillment and meaning in your life. People, in general, become fulfilled when they are working on something bigger than themselves.

And one of the many problems of short-term thinking is that it's very, very selfish. It's hard to think about others and things bigger than yourself if you're thinking about the next five minutes and the last five minutes.

And so part of the process of expanding your sense of time is you also expand your sense of who you are and what you are about.

If you can do that, you can find more meaning in your life because our own lives are so small and short that it's hard to find meaning in just them. We find meaning by connecting with something much larger than ourselves.

If we can become part of that, if we can see ourselves as an instrument, then we have become bigger, we have more meaning, and it's easier to become fulfilled.

I think that long-term thinking is healthy in many ways, and it's essential for society as a whole.

PRESTON SMILES

Personal Freedom Coach, member of ATL (Association of Transformational Leaders) founded by Jack Canfield, bestselling author of *Love Louder: 33 Ways to Amplify Your Life.*

I first came across Preston through his YouTube channel. He was musing about the mind, personal transformation, and philosophy. He had a talent for explaining big ideas in a way that was accessible and enjoyable. So I called him up to pick his brain.

The World You See, Is the World You Are

Duncan: When you talk about "the world you see, is the world you are," what do you mean by that?

Preston: I mean that we can't be separate from the filter. Everything is going through a filter.

We don't see, touch, taste, and hear the same.

For example, a tree. The landscaper sees the tree, and he goes, "Wow, it's so beautiful against the backdrop." Another person sees the tree, a botanist, and he's looking at the soil. Then I look at the tree, and I see my ancestors; I see the trees they hung from. Depending on the viewpoint from where you're looking, you will see and experience a different tree because everything is going through a filter. We cannot be separate from who we were raised by; we can't be separate from the TV we watched or the radio we've experienced.

We are constantly receiving; I think it's two million bits of information at any given moment, but we narrow that down because we would explode if we were actually receiving two million bits. So what we do is filter all that out and delete and distort the information so we can see what *we want* to see.

There was a study where they put cats in a room where everything was horizontal. *Everything* was horizontal. These cats were in this room for five months. Then they took them out and put them in another room where things were horizontal and vertical. The cats literally would just *boom* (crash into anything vertical, such as chair legs) because they had learned to delete and distort that information.

They had learned to only look in a particular way.

That is happening to us as well. So for me, it's about can we bring awareness to it because you cannot intervene in a world you cannot see.

A lot of people talk about "changing their lives," but they can't see what's been running them.

The Illusion Is That It's Easier Not to Care

Duncan: Why do you believe that separation is one of the biggest problems we have as a society?

Preston: When we believe we're separate, it's easier for us to hurt each other.

When we believe we're separate from nature, it's easier for us to frack and do a million other stupid ass things that hurt us in the long run, but we don't see it.

It's easier for us to say, who cares about tigers? Let them die off. We don't need tigers. We don't need lions. We don't need fish in the ocean; let's fish the hell out of them until we eat them all, and then screw it, maybe some more will pop up somewhere. The illusion is that it's easier not to care.

Have you ever seen somebody dancing their asses off at a party, and they suck, but they're just going for it? And you're like, "Yes! That dude is awesome!" On the reverse end, have you ever seen somebody get into an accident or run against a screen door or something, and you're like, "Ow," and you wince a little bit? That's your mirror neurons firing off. There's a part of all of us that is deeply connected. If we saw there was no separation, if we saw that all of this, that we're all playing together, we're all brothers and sisters, we're all deeply connected, then we would have to potentially care.

Life Is Just Life-ing

Preston: Stuff that we label good and bad. Those are mental constructs.

Life is impartial.

Life is just life-ing.

And we add these labels to it.

Whenever we can sort of pull out and have that bird's eye view, then we see that there is an order to the whole thing.

Responsibility

Duncan: Responsibility. This is a huge point. When we realize that we are responsible for our life, our first instinct might be fear. *Oh shit! Stuff I like, stuff I don't like, I am responsible for this?* But once you get over that hurdle, it is so exciting and empowering to think, *Hey, I can change or create anything that I want.* It's a big idea.

Preston: Yeah, it's pretty beautiful to realize that life isn't happening to you; it's responding to you. We are the authors, the sculptors, the painters, the Picassos of our life. And when we choose to do that by design instead of by default, we position ourselves to live an extraordinary life. Anybody who's ever lived an extraordinary life got that one thing. *It's up to me! If it's to be, it's up to me.*

However, responsibility is a tricky thing because many people say it, but not many people want to live from it. What responsibility looks like is really paying attention to everything you're experiencing now, like what's in your bank account? You're responsible for! What's happening in your family? You're responsible for! If I believe that part of it was you if I'm in the conversation of, "It's you, and I'm a victim to you," then you have my power and not me.

This could be a hard pill for some people to swallow because they get into the conversation of, "What about people in Africa and places where they don't have clean water and things of that nature?" It's the same thing. I've been in the bush in Tanzania with people who don't have clean water, and I would say the same to them. And interestingly enough, I'd say they are wealthier than most of the people I meet in the U.S. or the Western world.

Note: *Taking responsibility does not mean you're to blame for something.*

Challenging things happen all the time that are totally out of our control. Yet, we can take responsibility and ownership over how we act, think, and allow these things to define us.

The opposite mindset of responsibility is that of the victim.

When we believe we're a victim, there's always someone we can blame – politicians, the economy, Brexit, immigration, ex-husband, A.I., fill in the blank. This may provide temporary relief because we can point our fingers and get frustrated at something. But if we examine the terms and conditions, we'll realize that we've made a poor deal.

We have handed our happiness over to someone/something else, and we will forever be stranded out at sea, being blown about, helpless.

HELEN LAKELLY HUNT, PHD

Relationship expert, co-creator of 'Imago Relationship Therapy,' bestselling author, and philanthropist installed in the Women's Hall of Fame.

HARVILLE HENDRIX, PHD

Couples' therapist with more than forty years of experience, bestselling author of *Getting the Love You Want*, which Oprah described as "the best relationship book ever."

I was new to the work of Helen and Harville until a few days before interviewing them. But if Oprah describes your book as 'the best relationship book ever,' that's a good reason to do further research. It didn't take long to discover they are pioneers of human connection. For decades they have been transforming relationships all around the globe.

The Connection Is Ruptured

Harville: Full aliveness is a social experience. It comes only when you're *with* another who is significant to you and you're safe with that person.

It is like the baby at the beginning of life with a caretaker, babies who are not disturbed when they are born; we know that many babies are born in trauma. But if you come with a natural birth, there's a natural connecting with the caretaker. And if you look at babies and mothers, or babies and fathers, playing together even when babies have no language, there's a glee, a joy; that's who we are.

But something happens in that relationship with every child because parents don't know how to keep that going. They become interested in something else, and they don't know how to go back and keep the baby in the state of connecting. So the connecting is ruptured, and then it becomes a memory. But you remember you had it, and you remember that you lost it, and you want back what you lost. But you don't know how to get it back, so you cry, then the mother or father comes, and that may work, or you cry, and they don't come, then you cry some more, and then you quit crying because it didn't get them. But you keep trying to get that connecting going again. However, because we all have flaws as parents, it never becomes predictable and chronic. So it goes underground, and it shows up in adolescence, it shows up with your best friend, then it shows up when you fall in love, and when you're an adult.

We have millions of people who are engaging in the reconnecting process. When they get it back, they don't have psychological problems anymore. All psychological problems are functions of disconnection, and they're resolved when you connect.

Just Move from Judgment to Curiosity

Harville: About ten to fourteen percent of people in the Western world had relatively healthy childhoods. So the rest of us didn't, from minor to mild to severe. But just about everybody's walking around with a relational rupture from childhood, and they're trying to get it repaired.

Helen: Leonard Cohen, the musician, wrote, "There is a crack in everything. That's how the light gets in." It's where we're broken that the transformation, the beauty, can come if you know how to hold it and if you don't run from it.

Duncan: That reminds me of a Japanese aesthetic called wabi-sabi, which is about beauty in imperfection and impermanence. A person may have a vase, and it might be cracked, but rather than try and pretend the crack's not there, they would shine a spotlight on it and perhaps even gild it in gold. We're all cracked, we're all imperfect, and that's beautiful.

Harville: Our phrase for it is you accept 'Otherness.' The Other is not you. They are never going to be you. But all of us want the Other to be like us. "Why don't you be more logical and rational, then we wouldn't have all these problems," and she says, "Why don't you be more emotional, and then life would be more exciting." Well, we're not that! So we accept each other, and then the energy moves out of conflict into connecting and co-creating, and that's a total transformation of energy when you move it away from polarizing.

The deepest human need is to experience being with another person without criticism.

Couples don't know how to talk. In fact, hardly anybody knows how to talk without polarizing.

Because I usually think the world is the way I see it, it happens to be also the way you see it, but your view is wrong, and mine is right! So we have to learn how to talk so that we hold each other's separate realities, understand them, and accept them. We use the word *advocate* for your difference, advocate for your Otherness. So we advocate for you to be who you truly are with me. Even if it's sometimes at my discomfort because my discomfort simply means I have difficulty accepting difference.

But once I fully accept difference, then I don't have discomfort.

I have celebration for who you are and that I get to live with you, and that's a very different world than the struggle about who's going to run the show.

Helen: It's practicing shifting from judgment to curiosity. Judgment to curiosity and wonder, wonder about your partner.

I was a very accurate judge, I was right about my judgments of Harville, but we had a terrible relationship. So until I gave up judging him and just became curious and wondering more about him...

Harville: See, the thing is, when you hear Helen say this, it's so simple to have a great relationship. You move from judgment to curiosity.

We didn't make that up; this is the way it works. This is the way human beings work.

Helen: When you wonder about something and you're curious, you're put in the brain's dorsolateral prefrontal cortex. Neuroscientists say tolerating ambiguity is a sign of the best human brain health.

And when you're up here just wondering about your partner instead of judging them, all these neurochemicals of awe begin to course through your body.

If you can just let go of judging them and wonder about *why it is they think the way they think? Or feel the way they do?*

If you practice wonder, then you begin to be bathed in the neurochemicals of awe and wonder.

ARIELLE FORD

Relationship expert, bestselling author, and former president of the Ford Group, which helped launch the careers of Deepak Chopra, Jack Canfield, Mark Victor Hansen, and Neale Donald Walsch.

Hollywood films give us a pretty consistent model for what love looks like, but is that a helpful guide? Or are false expectations setting people up for failure? Our relationships affect our well-being, so I needed to know more about this.

Nine Irreconcilable Differences

Duncan: Research at the University of Washington has shown that every couple has a minimum, an absolute minimum, of nine irreconcilable differences. These are things which they're *never* going to agree on.

Arielle: Right, but we live life as if we should get along 24/7, not understanding that it's normal to have differences with people.

And the point of it is to learn how to be loving anyway and come up with creative solutions. One simple example: in every couple, generally you have a spender and a saver, totally opposing views about money. That's probably not going to change. But you can learn how to love and respect the other person's point of view and develop ways to negotiate how the money's being used and spent, so there's an understanding there.

Duncan: So the issue with these nine, at least nine, differences is people think, *Oh, there must be something wrong with my relationship,* and they end it because of the differences. As opposed to realizing this is normal. Do you think recognizing this will take a lot of pressure off people? *Arghh, okay, phew, this is normal for everyone.*

Arielle: We were all brainwashed with this "You meet your soul mate, fall in love, get married, and then live happily ever after." Yes, you meet, you fall in love; when you fall in love, your brain emits amazing, feel-good hormones like adrenaline, dopamine, and oxytocin. You are literally crazy in love. Or what I like to call the socially acceptable form of insanity.

But it only lasts for six to eighteen months. It's nature's trick to get us together, procreate, and keep making more humans.

But then you have to learn how to get along, and that's the stuff they never bothered to teach us in school. The real purpose of a soul mate relationship is to be a point of healing. You're with somebody who is your best friend, your lover, your safe place to land, and all your childhood issues, your childhood wounds can come up for healing. But you don't have to do it alone; you have this partner in life to do your healing with. That's the point of a true, committed relationship that somehow didn't get communicated to us.

JOHN GRAY, PHD

The bestselling relationship author of all time
with over 50 million books sold in more than fifty
languages throughout the world, author
of *Men Are from Mars, Women Are from Venus.*

*John has taught millions of individuals and couples
worldwide for more than forty-five years. USA Today listed
his book as one of the top ten most influential books of
the last quarter-century. His experience is unique, and
I was keen to hear his perspective on how humans connect.*

Testosterone Is Not the Villain

John: In the past, everybody's always associated irritation, annoyance, anger, violence, and aggression with high testosterone (in a man). But now science has told us it's not high testosterone – it's lack of confidence, not knowing what to do in a stressful situation.

For a man, self-esteem, confidence, and well-being come from testosterone. And testosterone's only produced when you earn something, when you do something, when you exert yourself, where you overcome something, that's testosterone. You lift a heavy weight; more testosterone gets produced. You get a light weight, sit at your desk all the time, do nothing; you don't build the testosterone.

The Testosterone Cycle

Duncan: Men naturally alternate between needing intimacy but then needing to back away and have autonomy and space. Can you give an example of how that might play out?

John: The tendency in the man – and in some women who are really on her male side – the testosterone tendency is you get close because you want to achieve a goal. You want intimacy. Intimacy and love, we all need it, we're all fulfilled through it, that's a human need – love, intimacy, closeness. So my testosterone gives me the motivation, the courage, the energy to connect.

So as I'm connecting, my testosterone's going up. I've achieved my goal, testosterone goes up, I'm feeling attracted and turned on if it's a sexual relationship, and then we connect. I've reached my goal. I've climbed the mountain.

Now I can relax.

Now my estrogen starts to go up.

I feel good about her. I feel good about me. I'm now experiencing intimacy; I'm now feeling this love. It's like when you're having sex, you say, "I just want to keep going forever," "I love you, I want this to be forever." That's addiction, that's attachment, estrogen is attachment.

So what's happening at that time is my testosterone's spiking and my estrogen's also spiking, so you're getting this elevated state of the whole spiritual being of testosterone and estrogen.

Then what happens is oxytocin gets released.

This oxytocin immediately pumps estrogen higher, which pushes your testosterone down. That's when you want to fall asleep.

As a man, you're in love with her, but that love is estrogen, and your testosterone's down. You need to pull away from her to be independent, autonomous, and on your own for a while. This will rebuild your testosterone.

And once your testosterone goes back up, your estrogen goes down.

Now you have your testosterone, you can achieve connection with her, and there's room for the estrogen to come back up.

And you connect.

Estrogen goes higher.

You've got to pull away.

So this is like this dance cycle between men and women always, where men get close, everything's good, then we need to pull away for a while to rebuild on our own.

Because there's nothing more delicious for a man than to feel, *Okay, I made this woman happy, I've fulfilled her. She's so happy to be with me.* You get the taste of that, and that's like a delicious coffee, you want more, it's like alcohol, you want more, it tastes so good, or drugs – I want more of that!

Now you're becoming too dependent, too attached.

And so there's a natural mechanism in men, which is your hormones trying to balance; you want to pull away, the body will start to pull away.

Many men don't understand this cycle; they don't give themselves permission to pull away. Remember I mentioned the man who didn't have a father? Or the man who had a father but the mother wasn't happy, and the father wasn't good. "Oh, your father's not here, your father didn't show up, he's not there, you can't depend on him." So what happens is the boy then feels guilty when he starts to pull away from the woman.

And the woman doesn't know men are supposed to pull away. When I pull away, my wife is relieved; she says, "Yeah, go out and be with your male friends," "Go chop wood," because she knows I come back more loving. She knows that's how I rebuild. Go to the gym, go out, go kayaking, ride your bike, write a book, get out there. Do something on your own to rebuild your testosterone. And chopping wood isn't the only way to do it; it's a fun metaphor, but literally, meditation is one of the ways I do it or driving. I drive my car and run some errands.

MADAN KATARIA, MD

Physician, founder of the Laughter Yoga
movement, over 20,000 laughter clubs
in 110 countries.

*"Laughter is the best medicine." I wanted to explore this
idea more. I've always thought of laughter as being
a byproduct of feeling amused. You feel happy or amused,
and that triggers laughter. But what would happen if you
flip the order around and put laughter at the beginning?
Madan Katara had this idea over twenty-five years ago,
and it started a movement.*

Motion Creates Emotion

Madan: Even if you laugh for the sake of laughing, even if you
act like a happy person, your body cannot tell the difference.

So I thought, if your body doesn't know the difference if you're
acting out, you could make laughter an exercise. That was the
breakthrough; we could fake it. We started faking laughter, and
within seconds, everybody was laughing for real.

In 1884, Professor William James, the father of psychology, hy-
pothesized that the bodily expression of any emotion could
reinforce that emotion in the mind. Even if you are acting like
a happy person from the body, it gives biofeedback to the mind,
and then your mind starts secreting the happy chemicals.

Same thing with depression. You're so upset, in turmoil, you can't think of doing anything. But you can do it from the body.

If you see depressed people, they walk slowly; they talk slowly, and their body movements are slower. If you change this around and move your body quickly and start laughing and playing, this resets in your mind.

This theory is called *motion creates emotion.*

We have a famous quote in laughter club: "We don't laugh because we are happy, we are happy because we laugh."

MICHAEL GREGER, MD

Physician, diplomat of the American Board of
Lifestyle Medicine, was invited to testify before
Congress, bestselling author of *How Not to Die.*

*I'd spoken to many specialists about the importance
of exercise for our mental health by this point. But
a question I didn't have an answer for was how does
exercise compare to prescription antidepressants?
I watch a lot of documentaries, and I started to
notice the same man's face popping up again and
again: Dr. Michael Greger. He was someone who had
researched this topic, so I gave him a call.*

Antidepressants vs. Exercise. Who Wins?

Duncan: There's so much evidence that exercise is correlated
with improved mental health, but what is the causal evidence
like at present?

Michael: That is an excellent question, so this is a perfect example of where you could imagine correlational evidence not
necessarily translating into causal evidence. For instance, you do
a cross-sectional study, a snapshot in time, and ask people, "Do
you exercise or not? Do you have symptoms of depression or not?"

And lo and behold, those people that exercise a lot will report
they have very low, on average, symptoms of depression.

And you say, "Awesome, exercise helps depression!"

Well, not so fast.

Maybe exercise leads to less depression, or depression leads to less exercise. You can imagine how if you're feeling crappy, you're not going to go out for a run, so maybe it's what's called *reverse causation*; perhaps it's the other way 'round.

And so what you need is this interventional study where you intervene and randomize people to different groups and see if you can actually help them. So that's what Duke University did; they randomized men and women over the age of fifty with major depression into one of two groups:

1) An aerobic exercise program for four months.

2) You take an antidepressant drug. In this case, it was Zoloft, one of the SSRIs, kind of a Prozac-like drug.

The way we measure depression is something called a Hamilton Depression score. So before exercise, people were up around eighteen, and anything over seven is considered depressed, so these are people who are severely depressed.

And within four months, the drug group came down to normal, which is what antidepressants are supposed to do; they're supposed to help depression.

But what happened to the exercise-only group, no drugs? They experienced the same powerful effect.

And so the researchers at Duke concluded, hey, exercise could be an alternative to antidepressants, given that they've shown it to be a feasible, effective treatment.

But critics of this study have pointed out that this was a group exercise program. People came in because if you say, "You exercise," "You don't exercise," how do you know they do it? And if nobody exercises, well, you've just wasted a lot of money doing a study. So, you had to come in three times a week to do a group class, and then we can make sure you're doing exercise.

Okay, but that adds a confounding factor; maybe the only reason the exercise group got better is because they're forced to get out of bed and interact with people.

Duncan: The connection of the group.

Michael: The social stimulation, and maybe it had nothing to do with the actual exercise. So before you could definitively say exercise works as good as these drugs, you need to do the same study, but you add a third group. They do exercise alone with no extra social interaction.

That's precisely what those same Duke University researchers did; they realized they could not get definitive answers until they had that third group. So they created what is, I believe, to date, the largest trial of exercise for people with major depression. And this wasn't just older adults but younger adults as well.

So they added this home exercise group. There was the supervised exercise group, the drug group, and then the home exercise group.

What happened?

They all worked just as well in forcing depression into remission.

So we can say now with confidence that exercise is comparable to antidepressant medication in the treatment of patients with major depression.

That was the biggest study, but there have been a number of them. You put all the studies together, and researchers have indicated that exercise has a large effect on reducing depression symptoms, calling it a powerful intervention.

Unfortunately, it's very rarely prescribed by doctors.

You go to a psychiatrist, and they're not going to tell you to buy running shoes. But they're also not going to get the kickbacks from the running shoe company as they may get from the pharmaceutical company.

Duncan: Is that the primary reason, or do you feel like it's at least moving in the right direction? Are doctors starting to prescribe it more?

Michael: A lot of it's ignorance. I don't want to paint doctors as being greedy with their handouts. There's just a lot of ignorance; they don't know about the power of simple lifestyle interventions like exercise to have these pharmacological-like effects. Doctors will say, "Well, of course, exercise is good for you, but it's actually going to help with major depression?" People are skeptical, but they're just not familiar with the evidence.

Side Effects

Duncan: You mentioned earlier the word *side effects*. Some of the side effects of antidepressants are sexual dysfunction – I think it affects around seventy to eighty percent of people – weight gain, insomnia, nausea, diarrhea. Exercise can achieve the same results as these antidepressants but without the harmful side effects?

Michael: I love that you said 'harmful' because exercise has got lots of side effects, but they're all good side effects. And so, not only is the exercise helping your brain; if that was all that it was doing, that's enough. But it's also increasing your cardiovascular health, improving your immunity, and doing all these other wonderful things to your body. That's the beauty of lifestyle medicine – you only get good side effects.

"Not exercising is like taking a depressant."

TAL BEN-SHAHAR, PHD

PETER RUSSELL

Physicist, bestselling author who predicted the internet in his 1982 book *Global Brain*, has been studying the mind, consciousness, and the core truth of spiritual traditions for over fifty years.

Each year Watkins magazine publishes a list of one hundred spiritual teachers, activists, authors, and thinkers changing the world. This is how I learned about the work of Peter Russell. Peter was a student of Stephen Hawking. He studied mathematics and theoretical physics at Cambridge University and then became fascinated by the mysteries of the human mind. He studied meditation and Eastern philosophy in India before returning and pioneering the introduction of human-potential seminars in the 1970s.

Searching and Aversion

Duncan: What do you feel are some of the most common things getting in the way of people being happy?

Peter: Yeah, it comes down to two labels.

One, there's the *searching*, and so many things come back to searching. It's the believing "If I just had something…got something…got some experience…I'd be happy." So that's a whole belief system.

The other one is almost the opposite, which is often called *aversion*. "If I just got rid of this," "Oh, if I just could get this person out of my life," or "get them to change," whatever it is, but there's something wrong in the world, there's something I don't like, and that's the other side of the coin.

They both boil down to the idea that if I can change the world somehow, either get something or avoid something; I'll be okay.

We then start treating people like objects. We treat them like going out for a good gourmet meal: "If this were on the menu, I'd be happy," "If my partner did this or said this, I'd be happy."

By Letting It In, We Get Freedom from It

Peter: I reframe 'letting go' as letting in and letting be.

It's not trying to get rid of something.

Say you've got some anger or grievance or something you're trying to let go of; instead of trying to get rid of it, which never works or seldom works, let the experience in.

If you're feeling anger, how does that feel in the body? Get to know the experience. What are the stories you're telling yourself about the person? Let that in, and then allow it to be there, not trying to get rid of it.

But what I find again and again is the more we bring our awareness to what's going on, it often just tends to dissolve of its own accord. You get the same thing when you do yoga. If you've got a tense muscle or a tight muscle that's not letting go, it's a battle if you try to make it let go. But people know if you tune into feeling that muscle, feeling the tension, allowing that experience of the tension in, then it often just relaxes of its own accord.

We're scared: *Oh, if I let this anger in, I will start swearing and spoil the relationship or lose my job,* or whatever. It's not about acting everything out but letting the experience in; one thing I do there for myself is, if I'm feeling like I've got some anger stuff or frustration going on, I'll write about it, and that is bringing it into awareness. I'll throw the paper away afterward; I'm not keeping a journal about it but just writing what I'm feeling. And I'll use language I won't even repeat on the internet! I'll write what I'm feeling: "Stupid blah blah blah blah blah," "What the blah do they think they're blah," and it's like, *Ahhh,* and I just feel so much better.

We keep things out on the edge of our consciousness; we don't let them in. "If I let this in, all hell will break loose."

In fact, by letting it in, we get freedom from it.

CHECKLIST REMINDER

1) FOUNDATIONS

I EAT WELL. I SLEEP WELL.

2) FUNDAMENTALS

A, B, C, D, E, F, G, H

I AM...

APPRECIATING

BEING

CONNECTING

DIRECTING

EXERCISING

FORGIVING

GROWING

HELPING

APPRECIATING

I am focusing on what I'm grateful and thankful for.

BEING

I am taking time to slow down, be in the moment, be still or anything that counteracts my constant 'doing.'

CONNECTING

I am spending time with people I love and am giving these relationships the energy and attention they deserve.

DIRECTING

I feel like I'm the director of my own life. I feel a sense of autonomy and choice.
NB: This is not to be confused with a futile attempt to control life or an obsession with certainty.

EXERCISING

I am moving my body and being active.

FORGIVING

I am forgiving myself for things I did/didn't do, and I am forgiving others. I am releasing shame, secrets, and resentment.

GROWING

I am developing, progressing, and growing each day.

HELPING

I am helping others and contributing to something larger than just myself.

CONCLUSION

We understand that if you are unhealthy and overweight, you need to eat a quality diet, move, and consume fewer calories. And most importantly, for this healthy living to become a lifestyle, something that is a consistent part of your life. This doesn't mean it has to be hard or boring; it just means it has to be there. If someone said all you need to do is eat three salads in one day and run until you collapse, then you're finished, and you'll be your perfect weight forever, we'd all know that was rubbish. It takes consistency to work; suggesting otherwise seems silly.

Even though this is so obvious with regards to our physical health, it's no different with our mental health and well-being. We can't binge on Oprah videos, meditate, and spend time with loved ones all in a twenty-four-hour window and then expect to be happy forever. It is about consistency and these habits becoming a part of your daily life.

My goal with this book was to demystify the subject of happiness and highlight practices and habits that are proven to make a difference.

I've done my best to provide evidence, scientific and anecdotal, as to why these habits are beneficial. But the only thing that will make a difference is if you do them.

If you forget ninety-nine percent of what you've read in this book, but you remember the checklist and make the eight habits part of your daily life. They will work even if you've forgotten why they work.

When I turned seventeen, I was allowed to start driving lessons. My friends who lived on farms had gone around the fields for years; they were comfortable behind the wheel, natural. I had no prior driving experience and was slow and awkward. But I turned up to each lesson and learned the instructions step by step. Despite not feeling like I was good, I passed my test the first time. Many of my friends were far better drivers than me, but they had picked up bad habits over the years and would fail test after test.

Bad habits = no driver's license

Good habits = driver's license

Bad life habits = unhappy

Good life habits = happy

In his book *Homo Deus*, Yuval Noah Harari says, "People just don't know what to pay attention to... In ancient times, having power meant having access to data. Today, having power means knowing what to ignore."

I hope this book allows you to ignore a lot of the convincing, contradictory, and overwhelming advice that we are bombarded with every day that not only doesn't increase our happiness but often makes us miserable.

Keep things simple. It's as easy as A, B, C...almost. Plus D, E, F, G, H.

AFTERWORD

The Tale of Two Wolves – A Cherokee Legend

An old Cherokee is teaching his grandson about life. "A fight is going on inside me," he said to the boy. "It is a terrible fight, and it is between two wolves. One is evil – he is anger, envy, sorrow, regret, greed, arrogance, self-pity, guilt, resentment, inferiority, lies, false pride, superiority, and ego."

He continued, "The other is good – he is joy, peace, love, hope, serenity, humility, kindness, benevolence, empathy, generosity, truth, compassion, and faith.

"The same fight is going on inside you – and inside every other person, too."

The grandson thought about it for a minute and then asked his grandfather, "Which wolf will win?"

The old Cherokee simply replied, "The one you feed."[15]

> **Note:** *Now that you know some causes of happiness and unhappiness, which one will you feed?*

MICRO-GOALS

This is not my idea. I've heard it described by various people in different ways over the years. But I'm a big fan of micro-goals: making goals so tiny that it's almost harder not to do them.

If you don't usually go to the gym, setting a New Year's resolution to go five times per week is probably not the best approach. If you only go four times one week, you feel like a failure, which is demotivating.

I like micro-goals because the focus is not on achieving outcomes and desired results but on building momentum and a feeling of progress.

An exercise micro-goal might be: I will do one push-up per day.

A learning micro-goal might be: I will read one page of a book per day.

If you want to start meditating, the micro-goal might be: I will take one deep inhale and exhale per day.

Now what happens in practice is if I'm doing one push-up, I might think, *Screw it, I'm already down here; I might as well do a few more.* The one page of the book I read might be pretty interesting, so I'll read another.

I have big goals and dreams also. But the way I create the habits and momentum that allow me to move closer towards them is by setting myself micro-goals that I consistently hit. That is how this book was written, through a micro-goal. I did not have to type a certain number of words per day or work for a specific time. My only goal was that each day, I would do something book-related. It could be writing a sentence, a single word, or even a comma. It didn't matter, but if I committed to doing something on the book every day, then at some point, a finished book would appear. It might not be a good book, but there would be a book!

In addition to the momentum that micro-goals create, they also boost self-confidence. You become someone who follows through and does what they say they will do.

The late Millard Fuller dedicated his life to serving the disadvantaged. He is credited for revolutionizing the concept of philanthropy and is the recipient of over fifty honorary degrees and the Presidential Medal of Freedom.

He said, "It is easier to act yourself into a new way of thinking than it is to think yourself into a new way of acting."

So with that in mind, use micro-goals or whatever your preferred method is to consistently act out the happiness habits described in this book. Then, the desired thinking will follow.

ACKNOWLEDGMENTS

Thank you so much to my family for being my biggest cheerleaders and support for all of my life.

Thank you to Marie, who has held my hand and guided me. Thank you for your friendship and for being brave enough to tell me that the first draft of the book was not good, neither was the second version...oh, and neither was the third.

Thank you: Farnoosh, Sahand, Raphael, and the magical place, the *Mezrab*. Those six months we spent training together were so special. I loved it, thank you!

Ally, thank you so much for adopting me while I started writing this book. The countryside, fresh air, lots of walks, and quiet were the perfect ingredients to embark on this project. You truly looked after me and were the most generous host. Watching terrible, low-budget Christmas movies with you was the perfect reward after a long day's writing.

Thank you to all my incredible friends, who have been amazingly supportive and have encouraged me from the very beginning. I am so lucky to have you in my life.

Clara, thank you so much for your assistance in editing the book. Your feedback has been fantastic. You have been a pleasure to work with, incredibly patient, and you've displayed dedication every step of the way.

Asia, as soon as I saw your portfolio, I knew I wanted the book interior to be designed and typeset by you. You're an incredible artist and have made this collaboration fun and easy. This project would be much worse off if not for you.

Max, I'm so glad to have met you. You're a great friend and unbelievably talented. Your belief in me, this project, and the larger mission have been unwavering. Your help has been invaluable. I couldn't hope for a better manager.

A big hug to Atuksha for a decade of awesome conversations, big ideas, and support. It's been fantastic and inspiring to have had a front-row seat to witness all you've achieved. I can't wait for many more decades of friendship.

Last but not least, this book is only possible because, for eight years, many of the most incredible minds in the world have agreed to give up their time and explain their ideas, their research, and their discoveries to me in layman's language. Their generosity has allowed us all to benefit from their collective wisdom, and I am forever grateful for this. It's been so much fun. I have learned and will continue to learn so much from you.

Thank you.

ENDNOTES

1   Soroka, Stuart. "Why do we pay more attention to negative news than to positive news?" LSE (blog), May 25, 2015, https://blogs.lse.ac.uk/politics andpolicy/why-is-there-no-good-news/

2   Altucher, James. "Ep. 18: James Altucher on Saying No, Failing Better, Business Building, and More." Podcast uploaded July 11, 2014. The Tim Ferriss Show, https://tim.blog/2014/07/11/james-altucher/

3   Pinker, Steven. "The media exaggerates negative news. This distortion has consequences." The Guardian, February 17, 2018, https://www.theguardian.com/commentisfree/2018/feb/17/steven-pinker-media-negative -news

4   The Darwin Project, "About The Darwin Project." Accessed circa. February, 2019, http://www.thedarwinproject.com/about/about.html

5   The Darwin Project, "Darwin's Unfolding Revolution." Accessed circa. February, 2019, https://www.thedarwinproject.com/revolution/revolution. html

6   László, Ervin. "Pre-Publication Readers' Comments about *Darwin's Unfolding Revolution* by David Loye". Accessed circa. February, 2019, http://www.thedarwinproject.com/revolution/book/prepub.pdf

7   Robbins, Tony. (This quote was taken from a Youtube video of Tony Robbins speaking, however the link is no longer active) Accessed circa. January, 2019, https://www.youtube.com/watch?v=SBgKfFX3uZE

8   Gawdat, Mo. Solve for Happy: Engineer Your Path to Joy. Gallery Books, May 2018. Page 229-230

9   Wolpert, Daniel. "The real reason for brains." TED Global, July, 2011, https://www.ted.com/talks/daniel_wolpert_the_real_reason_for_brain

10 Gawdat, Mo. Solve for Happy: Engineer Your Path to Joy. Gallery Books, March 21, 2017. Page 267